Organic All-Natural Products to Make at Home for Healthy Glowing Skin

Easy Homemade Vegan Cream, Lotion, Moisturizer, Body Butter, Makeup, Toner, Scrub, and Mask Recipes

Josephine Simon

Copyrights
All rights reserved. No part of this publication or the information in it may be quoted from or reproduced in any form by means such as printing, scanning, photocopying, or otherwise without prior written permission of the copyright holder.

Disclaimer and Terms of Use
Effort has been made to ensure that the information in this book is accurate and complete. However, the author and the publisher do not warrant the accuracy of the information, text, and graphics contained within the book due to the rapidly changing nature of science, research, known and unknown facts, and internet. The author and the publisher do not hold any responsibility for errors, omissions, or contrary interpretation of the subject matter herein. This book is presented solely for motivational and informational purposes only. The publisher and author of this book does not control or direct users' actions and are not responsible for the information or content shared, harm and/or action of the book readers.

The information herein is offered for informational purposes solely, and is universal as so. The presentation of the information is without contract or any type of guarantee assurance.

The information provided in this book is designed to provide helpful information on the subjects discussed. This book is not meant to be used, nor should it be used, to diagnose or treat any medical condition. For diagnosis or treatment of any medical problem, consult your own physician. The publisher and author are not responsible for any specific health or allergy needs that may require medical supervision and are not liable for any damages or negative consequences from any treatment, action, application or preparation, to any person reading or following the information in this book. References, if any, are provided for informational purposes only and do not constitute endorsement of any websites or other sources. Readers should be aware that the websites listed in this book, if any, may change.

ISBN: 978-1986690492

Printed in the United States

Contents

Introduction _____ 1
Why DIY? _____ 3
The Power of Plants _____ 9
What You Should Know _____ 13
Cleansers _____ 21
   Antibacterial Cleanser _____ 21
   Brightening Cleanser _____ 23
   Sensitive Skin Cleanser _____ 25
   Sulfur Soap Cleanser _____ 27
   Daily Greens Face Wash _____ 29
   Kombucha Cleanser _____ 31
   Clay Cleanser _____ 33
   Argan Oil Cleanser _____ 35
Exfoliators _____ 37
   Ayurvedic Scrub _____ 37
   Sensitive Skin Exfoliator _____ 39
   Mocha Scrub _____ 41
   Blackhead Buster _____ 43
   Rose & Chamomile Exfoliator _____ 44
   Acne Scar Scrub _____ 45
   Pink Scrub _____ 47
   Calendula Scrub _____ 48
Toners _____ 49
   Rosewater Toner _____ 49
   Goodnight Toner _____ 51
   Antioxidant Toner _____ 53
   Aloe Toner _____ 55
   Elderberry Toner _____ 57
   Acne Toner _____ 59
   Lavender Lemonade _____ 61
   Rosemary Rice Toner _____ 63

- Moisturizers — 65
  - Aloe Butter — 65
  - Eczema Cream — 67
  - Blue Moisturizer — 69
  - Lemon Butter — 71
  - Brightening Serum — 72
  - Frankincense and Myrrh — 73
  - Anti-Aging Eye Cream — 75
  - Acne Prone Moisturizer — 77
- Masks — 79
  - Rose Mask — 79
  - Papaya Mask — 81
  - Bentonite Mask — 83
  - Turmeric Mask — 85
  - Banana and Oats Mask — 87
  - Flaxseed Mask — 89
  - Matcha Mask — 91
  - Spirulina Mask — 93
  - Chocolate Mask — 95
  - Avocado Mask — 97
- Extras — 99
  - Lavender Makeup Remover — 99
  - Coconut Oil Sunscreen — 101
  - Cucumber Face Mist — 103
  - Anti-Aging Frankincense Night Oil — 105
  - Vanilla Lip Scrub — 106
  - Argan Aftershave Balm — 107
  - Super-Soothing Aftershave — 109
  - Spot Treater — 111
- Further Reading — 113
- Also by Josephine Simon — 115

Introduction

Whether you've been vegan for decades or are just now experimenting with the lifestyle, you may know that eliminating dairy, meat, and sugar from your diet helps to stabilize your insulin levels and hormones, which works wonders for acne. If you have aging or mature skin, you probably already know that a vegan diet is high in antioxidants and fatty acids that help prevent the early signs of aging all over your body, especially your face.

Now that you're sold on the power of plants as food, have you ever considered what they could do when applied directly to the skin? If plants have so many great compounds, shouldn't you be able to use them in skincare?

The answer is yes! Which is good news, because the vast majority of skincare products on the market are loaded with chemicals that add toxins to your body or even dehydrate your skin. In order to have healthy, glowing, acne-free skin, you need to work with your skin, not torture it with harsh chemicals. Fresh, all-natural skincare products, made for you and by you, work with your body's natural chemistry while taking full advantage of the power of plants!

There is a growing industry for plant-based skincare products, but they can be a little pricey. Why pay 50 dollars for a moisturizer when you could make it at home for a fraction of that? You might not have considered it before, but you *can* easily make your own vegan skincare products at home. It's easy, it's inexpensive, it's fun, and with correct storage it's also completely safe—much safer then chemical-laced store-bought products not suited to your unique skin profile. So what do you have to lose? Just products that are expensive and/or harmful for your skin and the environment!

Why DIY?

When there are so many skincare products on the market, you have to ask yourself, why even bother making them yourself?

Cost
There may be seemingly endless organic and vegan skincare products on the market, but that doesn't mean they're good for your wallet! Because people are becoming more aware of the benefits of a vegan diet and skincare regimen, the cost of these products is often exorbitant. This may leave you scratching your head wondering how simple ingredients like cocoa butter or pineapple juice could end up costing you so much.

Before a product makes it to your bathroom counter the ingredients have to be sourced, processed, and made shelf stable. This can be a complex process. Then the product has to be packaged, marketed, and distributed. Between the cost of packaging, marketing, and employee salaries from corporate to the factories, it becomes easy to see how vegan products can end up being so expensive.

If you want all the benefits of a vegan skincare regimen, without the cost, making your products yourself is your best bet. You only have to pay for the raw ingredients and invest 5–10 minutes of your time. Some of the ingredients, like essential oils or almond oil, may seem costly themselves, but with these ingredients, a little goes a long way. One bottle of an essential oil can be used time and time again to make dozens of different products, and not just for skincare—you can also put it in shampoos, toothpastes, and cleaning products for your house. When it comes to savings, buying in bulk is your best friend.

Safety

Oftentimes we assume that just because something is on the shelf in a skincare store or grocery store then it must be safe. But the skincare industry is actually not very well regulated, so that's not necessarily true.

Everyone has different skin and different allergies, so what is safe for one person might not be safe for another. Skincare companies don't usually alert you to this fact. For example, having chronic adult acne could be an indication of a food or chemical sensitivity. It could even indicate a severe allergy of which you're unaware. In fact, if you've suddenly had an unusual or severe acne flare-up, one of the first things you should do is get an allergy test, or at least eliminate the most common allergens from your diet.

However, cutting allergens out of your diet might not be enough. Plenty of common allergens, especially gluten, end up in skincare products. Check out the section on allergens to read more about common allergens that might be hiding in your store-bought skincare products.

Making your own products allows you to regulate safety and tailor the recipes to your skin's needs and sensitivities. Read on in this chapter to learn more about safely making skincare products.

Potency

You probably already know that when it comes to fruits and vegetables, the fresher they are, the better they are for you. This is true because valuable enzymes, vitamins, and other important compounds may break down or become less potent over time, especially when frozen, pasteurized, or mixed with chemicals.

The same is true when it comes to skincare. Would you rely on a can of veggies to get your nutrients? Probably not, so why would you expect a skincare product that has been sitting on the shelf for months or even years to deliver the benefits you need?

Because homemade skincare products contain the freshest ingredients, you can also expect them to be more potent, especially when it comes to fruits like pineapple and papaya that rely on enzymes for their skincare benefits.

Self-Empowerment
When it comes to your health, there's a lot of bad information and bad food out there. Struggling with acne, aging, or chronic dry skin can be really stressful, especially when you've tried seemingly everything. Rather than jumping from one product to another, take back control of your skin!

In order to protect yourself, you have to take control of the foods you eat and the products you put on your body. Making your own skincare products will require a little bit of study and experimentation so that you can better understand your skin and body overall. When you get more in tune with your body, you'll start to pinpoint acne triggers and identify which products work for you and which do not. Not to mention that being able to make things for yourself is a great feeling!

Better for the Environment
As mentioned above, one of the things that make skincare products so costly is packaging. Not only is that a cost you don't want to have to pay for, but most packaging is bad for the environment. Every time you throw away a bottle, box, or jar, it just ends up in a landfill. When you make your own skincare products you eliminate the environmental costs because you're not using disposable packaging that just ends up polluting our precious natural environment.

There are lots of ways that non-organic skincare products can be bad for the environment. Microbeads are little balls of plastic often used in exfoliators. You probably don't want to rub tiny pieces of plastic against your skin, and you *definitely* don't want them washing down the drain. Microbeads are so bad for the environment that they've even been banned in the UK, the Netherlands, and several other European countries, and many organizations have called for a worldwide ban. In the US, a microbead ban began in 2017 and will take full effect in 2019.

So why are microbeads so bad? Once you exfoliate your face or body with microbeads, hundreds of thousands of tiny plastic beads wash down your drain. These pieces of plastic are too small to be filtered out, so they end up in bodies of water. Microbeads are very absorbent, so they absorb and transport dangerous toxins. Marine creatures, especially oysters, then consume these toxic microbeads. Sometimes the microbeads kill marine life, other times the marine life is eaten by a human and the toxins are introduced into the body. It's a dangerous cycle.

When you make your own exfoliators, there is no need to use microbeads. Pineapple, apple cider vinegar, oats, rice, and nuts can all serve as alternative exfoliants.

You may already be familiar with the environmental harms of non-organic farming. Fertilizers and other toxic chemicals end up in the water supply and seep deeply into the earth. It's still unclear exactly what repercussions non-organic farming will have on the earth and future populations, but using imagination, common sense, and scientific studies, you can be sure that it isn't good.

If you aren't already using organic skincare products, you may be buying into an industry that is clearly polluting our earth's fragile ecosystem. If you're using skincare products laced with chemicals, you also need to remember that when you wash your face, these harmful chemicals wash down the drain and end up in the water supply and the soil.

The best way to make your skincare products as ecofriendly as possible is to use organic ingredients and store them in recycled containers. Mason jars and recycled food jars, are all good options; just make sure to thoroughly sanitize (not just wash) your storage containers before use.

Gifts
What do you get for the person who has everything? Something thoughtfully handmade! Homemade skincare products let you save money on gifts while giving your friends and family a personalized, ecofriendly present to suit their tastes and needs.

The Power of Plants

If you've already converted to a vegan diet but haven't made the switch with your skincare, not only are you still introducing toxins into your body, but you are also missing out on the full power of plants!

The recipes in this book are quick and easy to make and require just a few ingredients. They also don't call for any special equipment you wouldn't already have in your kitchen.

Check out some of these plant ingredients and how they can add to your skincare regimen. All of these ingredients can be easily found at the grocery store or health food store, and all of them are listed in some of the recipes in this book.

Coconut Oil
Coconut oil is loaded with saturated fats (the good kind). This works wonders for trapping moisture in the skin. Since it also delivers balanced moisture to the skin, coconut oil can make for a great night cream if you're prone to dry skin or are worried about aging. It will also save your face in the winter (literally)!

Too many face washes on the market strip your skin of its natural oils while delivering harsh chemicals to your pores. This can cause acne and an overproduction of oil, forcing you to turn to harsher and harsher face washes—a terrible cycle. Coconut oil is antimicrobial, making it an effective acne treatment. Coconut oil is also a good choice as a carrier oil when applying stronger oils, like tea tree or manuka essential oils, to the skin.

As an added bonus, coconut oil has some natural SPF and can be very soothing on sunburns. Good news for sun worshipers!

Pineapple

Not only is pineapple rich in vitamin C, it also provides an important enzyme called bromelain. When reading about skincare or browsing the skincare aisle, you'll probably see alpha hydroxy acid (AHA) come up. AHAs are often used to exfoliate skin, reduce sun damage, reduce inflammation, unclog pores, and reduce the appearance of wrinkles. Unfortunately, most AHA products are chemical-heavy and totally artificial. This is where pineapple comes in.

Bromelain is a type of AHA that dissolves protein, making it the perfect exfoliating tool. Exfoliation is necessary in any skincare routine, especially if you have acne or acne scars, but many exfoliators on the market are too harsh to be truly helpful. Pineapple is the perfect solution. Papaya is likewise rich in bromelain.

Rose hip Seed Oil

Rose hip seed oil is high in two vitamins needed for skin health, vitamin A and vitamin C. Vitamin C prevents photodamage, while vitamin A increases collagen production. Both deliver antioxidant benefits, like fighting inflammation and reducing free radicals. Including vitamin A and C in your skincare routine will lead to glowing skin. Rose hip seed oil is also high in essential fatty acids, so it can help prevent signs of aging. Using rose hip seed oil can help to heal sun-damaged skin and reduce the appearance of acne scars and wrinkles. Oh, and it smells great!

Activated Charcoal

Activated charcoal is a powerful way to filter toxins. It's used in water filtration systems and even in hospitals to help those who have ingested poison. Integrating activated charcoal into your skincare regimen can bring those same detoxifying effects to your face. Activated charcoal will literally bind to any toxins in your skin and get rid of them. Bamboo charcoal is especially popular in skincare products. Wash your toxins away with activated charcoal!

Argan Oil

Argan oil is grown only in Africa and has a delicious nutty flavor that makes it hard to resist. Argan oil is loaded with vitamin E and fatty acids, and it absorbs into the skin easily, making it an ideal way to moisturize. Argan oil is also rich in antioxidants, delivering an anti-aging and anti-inflammatory effect. Because of its natural moisturizing and anti-inflammatory effects, it's a great choice for skin that is acne prone yet dry.

For some reason, a lot of men think scents like lavender and rose are too feminine for them. They're definitely missing out! But argan oil is considered a gender-neutral fragrance, so it's often used in products for men. Making a gift for one of your guy friends or family members? Try adding argan oil.

Bentonite Clay

If you're struggling with acne, drop everything and start using bentonite clay. Really—do a quick internet search for before-and-after pictures. This clay is seriously powerful. Not only is it loaded with minerals, it also sucks your pores clean and binds to toxins, effectively washing them down the sink. You can literally feel the sucking action; a mask made from bentonite clay will make your face pulsate. It also increases blood flow to your face, which helps in healing acne and acne scars. Be aware, though, that it can make your face red for about 30 minutes after use, so it might be best to use this clay at night.

Tea Tree Oil

Tea tree oil is another seemingly magic ingredient that can work wonders for your skin. It's extracted from the melaleuca shrub traditionally cultivated in Australia, where Aboriginal people have been using tea tree oil for centuries. Tea tree oil is beloved in acne treatments in part because of its incredible antiseptic effect. It also has an anti-inflammatory effect, cleans pores, literally dries out pimples, and unclogs oil glands, so it's a great choice for cystic acne. Additionally, tea tree oil is said to help diminish the appearance of acne scars.

Apple Cider Vinegar
Apple cider vinegar (ACV) is a must in any vegan pantry. Not only does it help out in vegan baking, it's also great in cleaning products, including the ones you use on your face. Like pineapples and papayas, ACV is high in AHAs, so it helps to dissolve dead cells, making it useful in fighting acne as well as hyperpigmentation. It also contains malic acid, which is antibacterial and can help reduce the appearance of acne scars. ACV makes a good base for toners and a powerful addition to a face masks, fighting acne and discoloration while balancing your skin's pH levels.

What You Should Know

If you're new to the *au naturel* skincare journey, there are a few things you should know.

Detoxing
When you begin the process of detoxifying your body and skin, whether through a vegan diet, all-natural skincare products, or both, your skin might freak out a little. Breakouts are a totally normal part of detoxifying, as the toxins are being released from your muscles and skin back into your bloodstream to be filtered out.

If you start breaking out because of these products or a vegan lifestyle change, don't worry. It actually means the products are working. Amp up your water intake, hit the sauna or a hot yoga class, get a massage, and prepare to have glowing, beautiful skin in the coming weeks or months.

Breakouts aren't the only symptom of an effective detox. With major lifestyle changes you may even begin to experience flu-like symptoms. Persist in your endeavor to clean up your life and you should see major changes in your health and skin Remember that your skin reflects your internal health!

When to See a Doctor
If breakouts persist, however, it could be a sign that you're eating or using a product you're allergic to. It's recommended that those with persistent acne seek medical help. Past your teenage years, acne is usually a sign from your body that something is wrong. It could be that you're facing a food sensitivity. Adult acne could also indicate hormonal issues or high stress levels, so if you continue to suffer from acne, speaking to a doctor or holistic

healer can really help. Some people even swear by acupuncture treatments for clearing up their acne.

Allergies

Using products to which you're unknowingly allergic could be causing rashes, dry skin, redness, inflammation, hives, and even chronic acne. Check out this list of common allergens often found in skincare products that might be irritating your skin. If you're struggling with any of these issues, look at the ingredients in your skincare products to see if any of these allergens might be lurking in the products you're rubbing on your face every day.

- **Gluten**—Those sensitive or intolerant to gluten should also avoid gluten in skincare products. Sadly, many products on the market contain gluten as a filler ingredient. Using products with gluten can cause rashes, irritation, and even hair loss! If you are gluten sensitive, making your own products at home is a safe bet. None of the recipes in this book contain gluten, assuming you use gluten-free oats.
- **Acid**—Acids used in skincare are designed to remove dead skin cells, an important part of any skincare routine. However, synthetic acids can cause redness, rashes, and irritation. Instead of using harsh synthetic chemicals, try natural fruit enzymes like those found in apples, pineapples, and papaya, as well as those found in herbs like white willow bark.
- **Synthetic Fragrance**—You may love the smell of your moisturizer, but the chemicals used to create the scent might be causing your skin problems. Allergic reactions to synthetic fragrances could cause rashes, hives, irritation, and dryness, as well as headaches, dizziness, watery eyes, a runny nose, and respiratory issues. The recipes in this book do not call for fragrances; instead, the essential oils used for their skin benefits provide a subtle and

calming fragrance with none of the chemicals. Not all fragrances are right for everyone, though. Before you make a skincare product with an essential oil you've never used before, make sure you don't find the scent off-putting. You should also check to make sure you won't have a bad reaction to a new oil. Mix a few drops of oil with a carrier oil, like coconut or olive, and put a few drops on your hand. If there is no reaction after a few hours, you're good to go. You should also keep in mind that not all essential oils are created equally. Since you'll be putting these oils on your face, it's worth it to invest in high quality, medical grade essential oils.

- **Emollients**—Emollients are often added to skin care products to help them go on more smoothly. Emollients may make products smoother, but they can also trigger acne, clog hair follicles, and cause boils, rashes, and overheating. Yikes! All-natural oils go on smoothly enough without irritating your skin.
- **Parabens**—Parabens are a class of artificial preservatives used in skincare products. Take a look at your skincare products and see if there are any parabens in them. They may be listed as butyl-, methyl-, and propyl-paraben. The jury is out on how unsafe parabens are, but it seems that pregnant women, at least, should avoid them. If you do have a sensitivity to parabens, it might cause rashes. None of the recipes in this book call for artificial preservatives. Most vegans try to avoid artificial preservatives whether in food or skincare products.
- **Sulfates**—In commercial products, sulfates are used to cleanse skin and create a foamy lather. However, sulfates can actually be dehydrating for the skin. They may also leach the color from dyed hair. Oils, clay, and apple cider vinegar can all replace the cleansing action of sulfates, while soapwort oil can create a lathering, soapy action.

- **Tree Nuts**—Nuts are a common allergy. However, not everyone who is allergic to eating nuts is allergic to using them on their skin—and vice versa. Nuts may come up even in organic skincare products as exfoliants, sweet almond oil, and coconut oil. Many of the recipes in this book *do* call for tree nuts. If you are concerned that you may have a sensitivity, spot test the recipe by putting a small amount on your arm or hand and waiting to see what happens. If you do find that you have a nut allergy, replace sweet almond oil or coconut oil with any of the other oils in this book. If you're on a budget, you can even use olive oil. If a recipe calls for nuts as an exfoliant, replace the nuts with rolled oats or rice.

Safety

Many of these products will need to be covered and stored in the refrigerator. The recipes in this book will indicate which need to be refrigerated. Also keep in mind that if a recipe calls for fresh fruits and veggies, you should only continue using the product as long as you would keep eating it if it were food. These products will often tell you when they are no longer safe to use. Mold growth and funky odors will indicate when you should definitely stop using a product, so you shouldn't worry too much about that.

When making your skincare products at home, it's best to use equipment you've set aside for that purpose. The only equipment you'll need for these recipes are spoons, bowls, a food processor, and storage containers. If you don't want to buy new equipment for your DIY skincare products, that's OK. You just have to make sure to sterilize the equipment before you use it. More on that later.

To be as ecofriendly as possible, you should use reusable storage containers. Glass jars, whether purchased or recycled, are best. Reusing food jars prevents them from ending up in a landfill. Like the equipment, you just have to make sure to sterilize your containers as well.

Sterilization

Sterilization is necessary, especially with all-natural products, because these recipes don't call for any preservatives Sterilization is not the same thing as washing. Just because something looks clean doesn't mean that it actually is, because you can't see all of the bacteria, fungi, and yeast that may be lurking. Failing to sterilize could mean that your products grow mold and don't last as long. It could also mean that bacteria grow without you noticing—not something you want to rub on your face! Here are two easy ways you can sterilize glass jars or kitchen equipment.

- **Dishwasher**—A dishwasher can be used to sterilize glass jars if it has a steam wash, sterilize, or high temperature setting.

- **Microwave**—Microwaving can kill the bacteria and other contaminants, but this method won't work if there's any metal on the jar. Just wet the jar slightly and microwave for 45 seconds. Do not put anything metal in the microwave, unless you want to witness an explosion in your kitchen!

Note: *Do not add cold liquid to a hot jar or vice versa. This could cause the jar to shatter, harming you in the process.*

Keeping a journal

If you're struggling from chronic acne, one of the best things you can do is keep a journal.

In your journal you should record what you eat each day, in detail, as well as which products you use on your skin. Be sure to list what ingredients are in each product. You should also describe how your skin feels each day in lots of detail. Did you have a breakout? How many spots? How long did they last? Were they cystic? You can also include information about stress levels, emotional health, skin texture, and dryness.

For women, indicate when you are menstruating or even keep a menstrual calendar. Do you see worse breakouts when you are about to get your period?

Reviewing the information in your journal can help you to draw connections between acne and possible hormonal, emotional, or food triggers. This will also help you to make sure that the homemade, vegan skincare products you're using are safe for you.

If you end up seeing a dermatologist, acupuncturist, nutritionist, or holistic healer to get your skin issues under control, this is information they're going to ask you for anyway, so starting a skin journal now can save you a lot of time in the future.

Other Thoughts
Did you know your skin is your body's largest organ? It's also your body's protective shield against the world, preventing bacteria, toxins, and UV rays from entering your body. This means it's of paramount importance to take care of your skin health in order to ensure the overall health of your body.

Your skin is already busy processing all of the toxins and pollutants that the outside world throws at it, so you don't want to add any more into the mix with your skincare regimen.

Unlike most skincare products on the market, the recipes in this book are not one size fits all, which is an erroneous concept when you really think about it. Instead, you'll have to experiment to see which recipes work best for you and how much to use.

Because of that, it's hard to estimate how many uses each recipe will yield, or how much you should use. The amounts listed are just a guideline. You should empower yourself to experiment and find the best solutions for you. If you tend to use products in smaller amounts, reduce the measurements in the recipes so you don't contribute to food waste.

These recipes also aren't set in stone. Don't like the smell of lavender? Replace it with another soothing, anti-inflammatory essential oil, like Roman chamomile or pomegranate seed oil. Feel free to steer away from the guidelines and make these recipes your own. You are the only person in your skin, after all, so only you know what's best for you.

Cleansers

Antibacterial Cleanser

Cleansing Castile soap combined with lavender and tea tree oils make this cleanser a powerful but gentle way to kill the bacteria that cause acne.

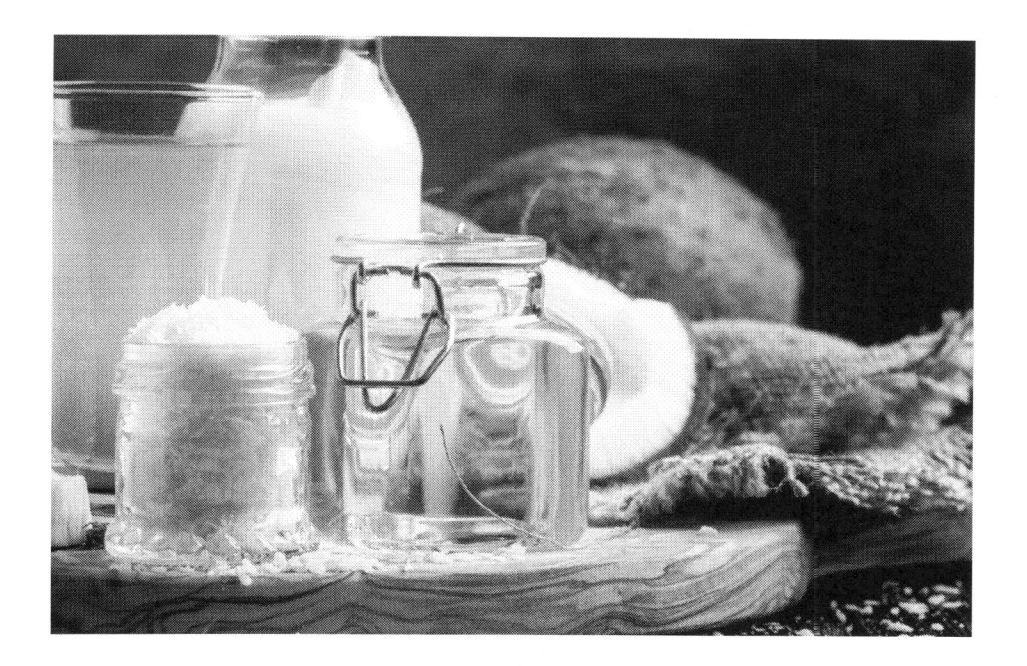

Ingredients

1 cup coconut water
¼ cup Castile soap
5 drops tea tree essential oil
5 drops lavender essential oil

Preparation

1. Mix all ingredients together and store in a bottle or foam dispenser if you want a foaming face wash.

Storage
1. Store this product in an airtight container in the refrigerator for up to a week.

Directions for Use
1. Shake well before use.
2. Use once or twice a day to cleanse your skin. Wet face with warm water and rub in cleanser in circular motions.
3. Rinse off and follow with an all-natural toner and moisturizer.

Brightening Cleanser

Rice powder has been used by women in Asia for centuries to create glowing, smooth skin. Brightening essential oils and gentle exfoliation from the rice powder make this cleanser a great choice for mature and sensitive skin.

Ingredients
¼ cup sweet almond oil
3 tablespoons rice, ground
5 drops sandalwood essential oil
2 drops lavender essential oil
1 drop lemongrass essential oil

Preparation
1. Grind the rice into a fine powder in a blender, coffee grinder, or food processor.
2. Mix the ground rice with the oils and combine well.

Storage
1. Store this product in an airtight container.

Directions for Use
1. Shake well before use.
2. Use once a day to cleanse your skin. Wet face with warm water and rub in cleanser in circular motions.
3. Rinse off and follow with an all-natural toner and moisturizer.

Sensitive Skin Cleanser

When you have sensitive skin it can be nearly impossible to find a cleanser that works for you. This cleanser is super gentle, with a unique blend of essential oils that soothe your skin *and* your mind.

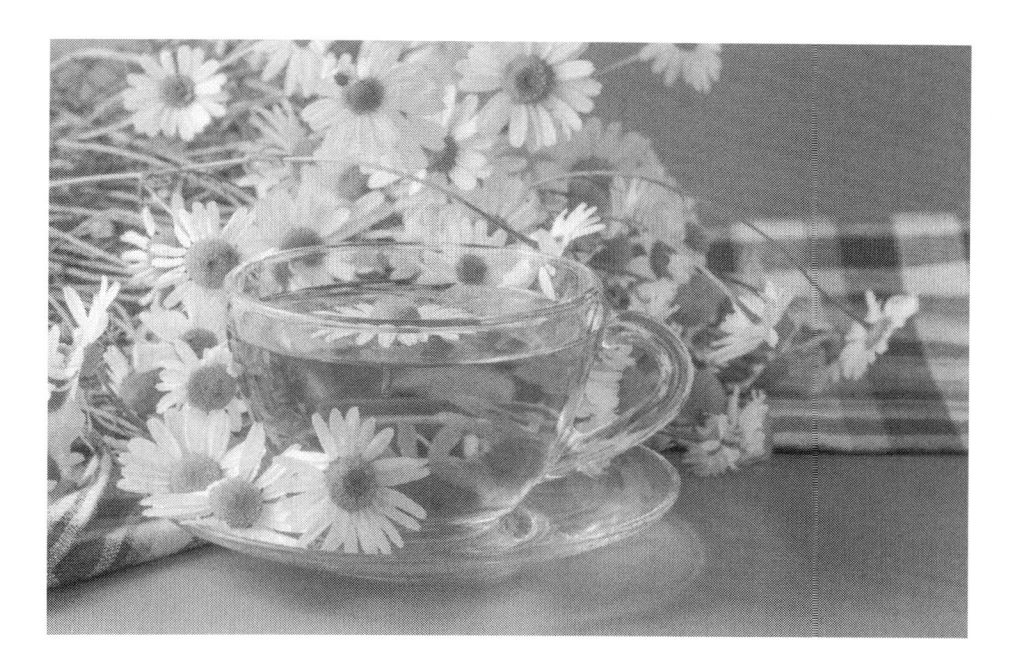

Ingredients
1 cup chamomile tea
¼ cup aloe vera gel
1 tablespoon soapwort extract
2 tablespoons jojoba oil
6 drops ylang ylang essential oil
5 drops lavender essential oil
2 drops cedarwood oil

Preparation
1. Mix all ingredients together, making sure to combine well.

Storage
1. Store this product in an airtight container in the refrigerator for up to one month.

Directions for Use
1. Shake well before use.
2. Use once a day to cleanse your skin. Wet face with warm water and rub in cleanser in circular motions.
3. Rinse off and follow with an all-natural toner and moisturizer.

Sulfur Soap Cleanser

Sulfur is probably not the first thing you would think to put on your skin, but this naturally occurring element can tackle acne by killing bacteria and regulating oil production. It might not smell great, but some people with acne prone skin swear by it. Both sulfur and African black soap have been said to work wonders for acne prone skin.

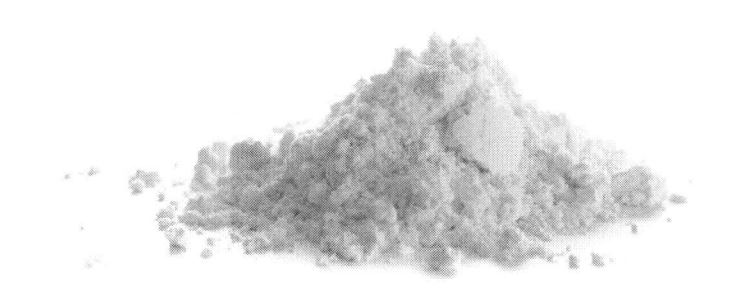

Ingredients
1 cup water, boiling
¼ cup African black soap, grated
2 tablespoons aloe vera gel
2 tablespoons argan oil
1 tablespoon sulfur powder
1 teaspoon vitamin E oil
10 drops lavender oil

Preparation
1. In a large bowl, mix together African black soap and boiling water until soap is dissolved.
2. Add in remaining ingredients and store in a soap dispenser or bottle.

Storage
1. Store this product in an airtight container in the refrigerator for up to one month.

Directions for Use
1. Shake well before use.
2. Use once a day to cleanse your skin. Wet face with warm water and rub in cleanser in circular motions.
3. Rinse off and follow with an all-natural toner and moisturizer.

Daily Greens Face Wash

You know you have you eat greens every day for your body, but what about greens every day for your face? These green superfoods are incredibly high in antioxidants, so they can reduce inflammation as well as the signs of aging.

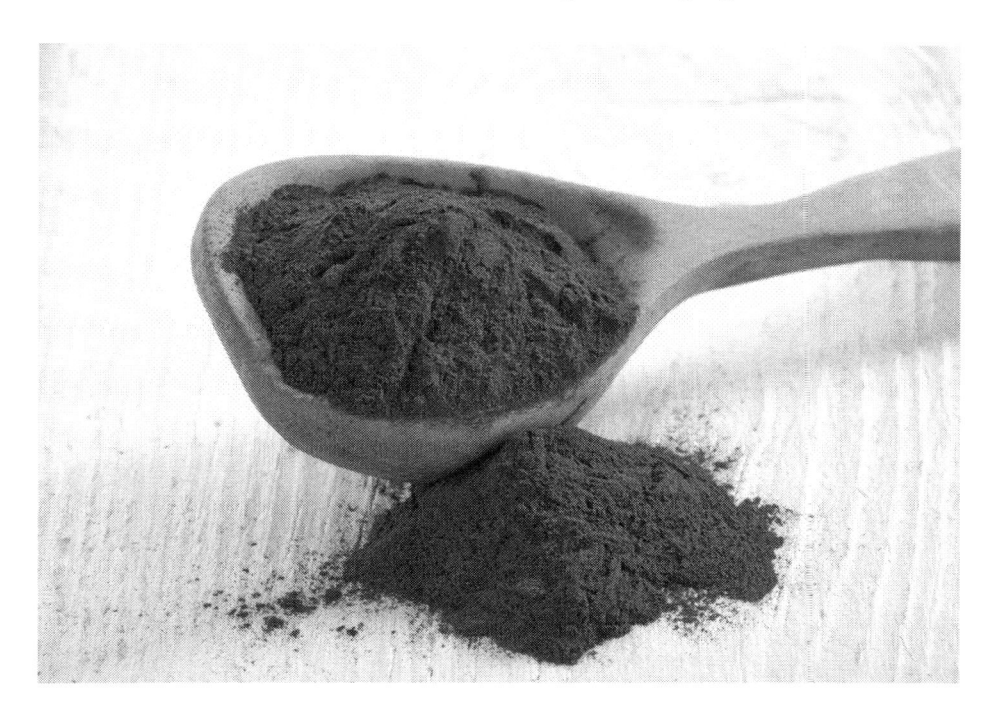

Ingredients
1 cup water, hot
2 tablespoons French green clay
2 tablespoons avocado oil
1 tablespoon soapwort extract
1 teaspoon matcha powder
1 teaspoon spirulina powder

Preparation
1. Mix all ingredients together and pour into an airtight container once cool.

Storage
1. Store this product in an airtight container in the refrigerator.

Directions for Use
1. Shake well before use.
2. Use once a day to cleanse your skin. Wet face with warm water and rub in cleanser in circular motions.
3. Rinse off and follow with an all-natural toner and moisturizer.

Kombucha Cleanser

Kombucha is a kind of fermented tea that is filled with probiotics that are great for your gut health. It's also reported to have brightening and anti-aging effects when rubbed on the skin, and it contains naturally occurring alcohol that kills bad bacteria. Whether you drink it or rub it on, it's great for skin! Wanna take your vegan cred up a notch? You can even make kombucha in your own kitchen rather than buying it at the store (where it can be a tad pricey).

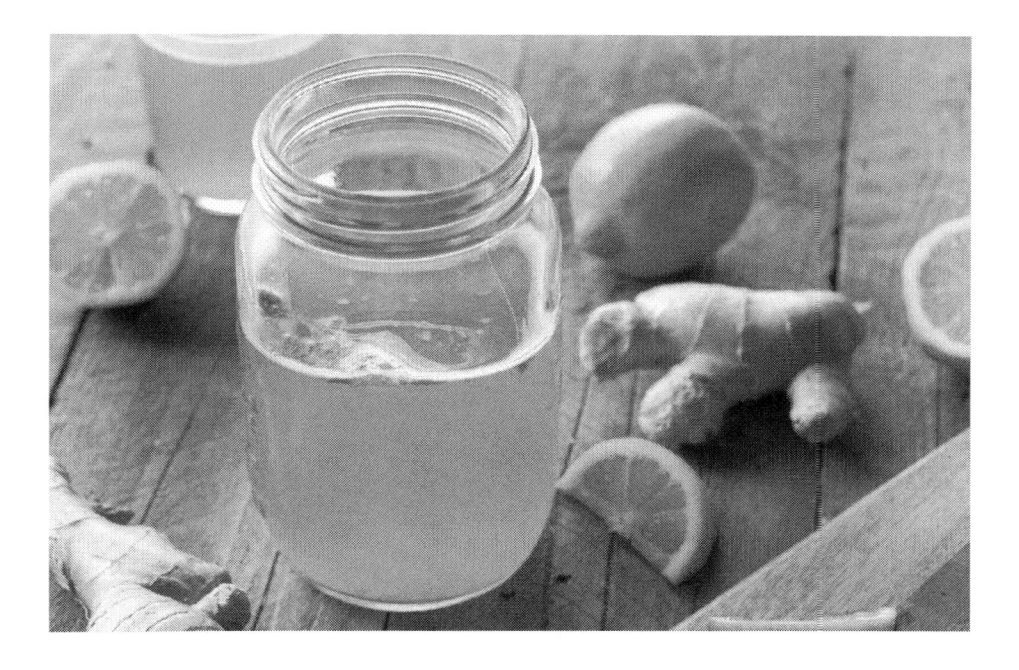

Ingredients
¾ cup kombucha
¼ cup Castile soap
2 tablespoons jojoba oil
5 drops geranium essential oil
2 drops grapefruit essential oil

Preparation
1. Mix all ingredients together and pour into an airtight container.

Storage
1. Store this product in an airtight container in the refrigerator. Because kombucha is fermented, it doesn't really spoil; it will just take on a more sour taste and smell over time.

Directions for Use
1. Shake well before use.
2. Use once or twice a day to cleanse your skin. Wet face with warm water and rub in cleanser in circular motions.
3. Rinse off and follow with an all-natural toner and moisturizer.

Clay Cleanser

Women have been using clay as a skincare product for centuries, if not thousands of years. Moisturizing, exfoliating, cleansing, this ancient skincare secret is sure to deeply cleanse your skin.

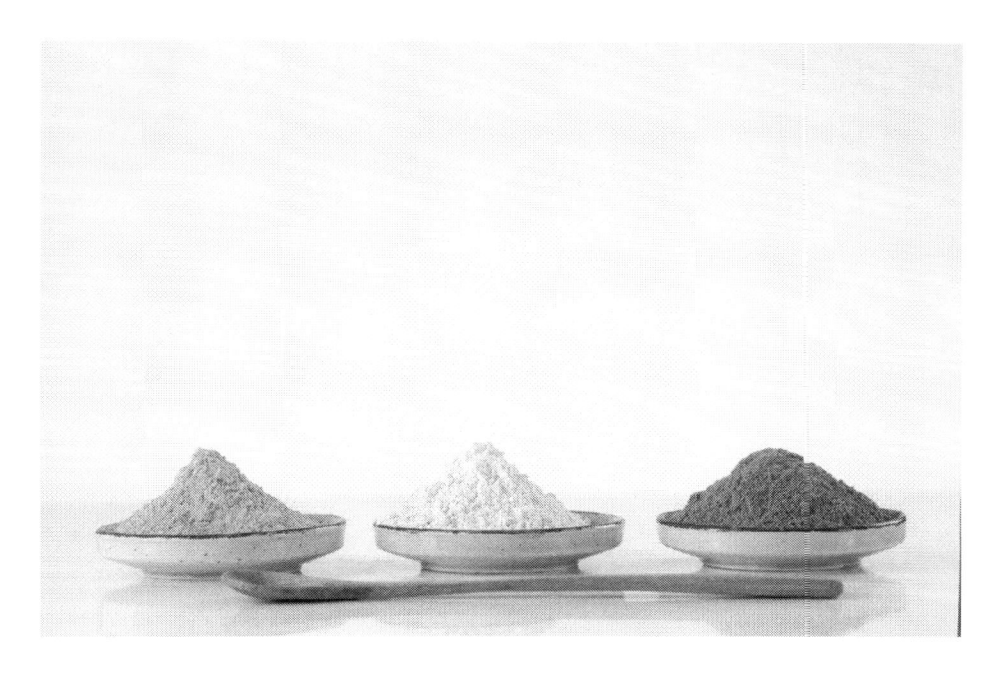

Ingredients
1 cup coconut water
¼ cup Castile soap
1 tablespoon rose clay
1 tablespoon white kaolin clay
1 tablespoon bentonite clay
3 drops lavender essential oil
3 drops patchouli essential oil
3 drops sandalwood essential oil

Preparation
1. Mix all ingredients together and pour into an airtight container.

Storage
1. Store in an airtight container.

Directions for Use
1. Shake well before use.
2. Use once a day to cleanse your skin. Wet face with warm water and rub in cleanser in circular motions.
3. Rinse off and follow with an all-natural toner and moisturizer.

Argan Oil Cleanser

Argan oil delivers a killer moisturizing effect, while antibacterial fractionated coconut oil deeply cleanses pores.

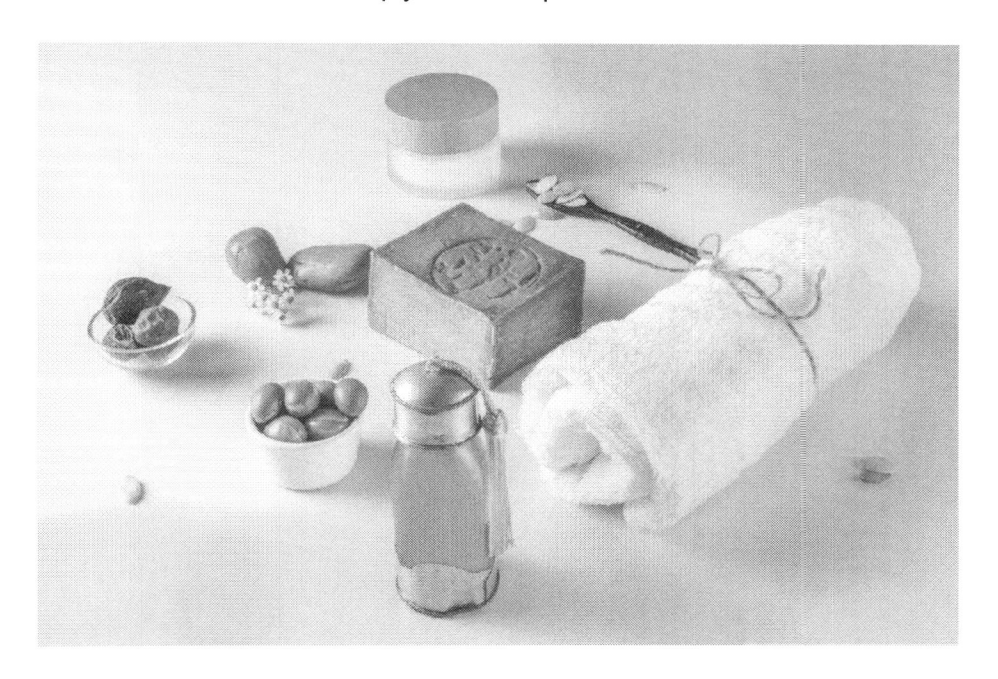

Ingredients
½ cup fractionated coconut oil
¼ cup argan oil
10 drops carrot seed oil
10 drops rose hip seed oil

Preparation
1. Mix all ingredients together and pour into an airtight container.

Storage
1. Store this product in an airtight container.

Directions for Use
1. Shake well before use.
2. To use, pour some of the oil on a cotton pad and rub on face until clean. No need to rinse with water, but you can use a toner after if you feel greasy.

Exfoliators

Ayurvedic Scrub

Ayurveda is the yogic science of healing and nutrition. The ancient practice is also the best kind of holistic anti-aging regimen. This scrub is anti-inflammatory, healing, and great for acne.

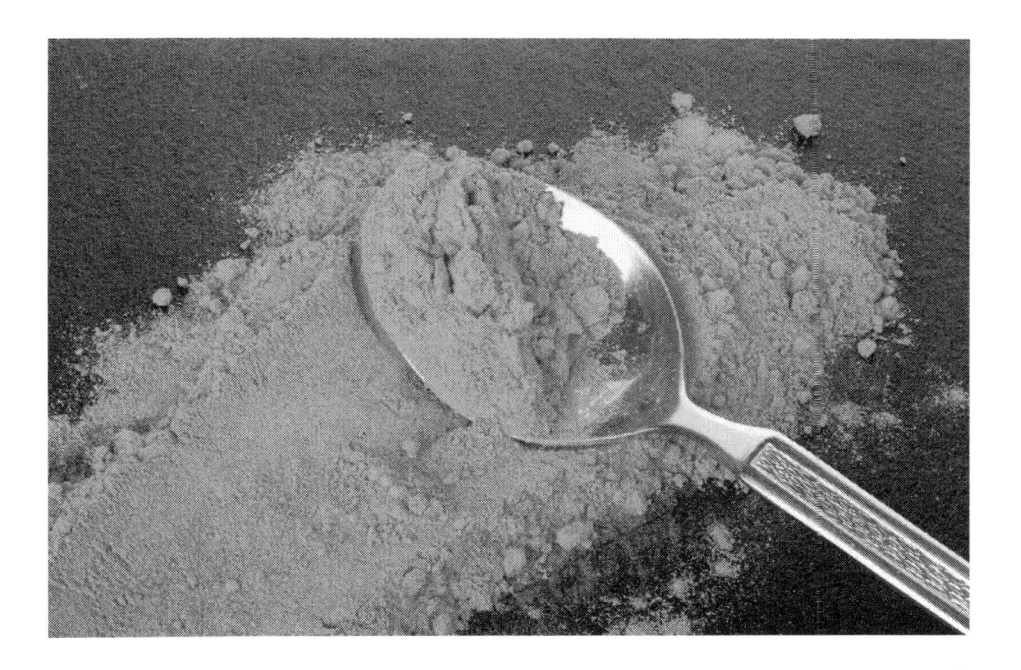

Ingredients
2 tablespoons coconut oil, melted (or fractionated coccnut oil)
2 tablespoons rolled oats
1 teaspoon turmeric powder
1 teaspoon lemon juice, fresh (optional)
10 drops neem oil

Preparation
1. Make sure the coconut oil is melted, but not hot—you don't want to cook the oats. Coconut oil usually melts at room temperature, so you probably won't have to heat it at all. Soak the oats in the melted coconut oil.
2. Mix in the rest of the ingredients.
3. Turmeric can stain your equipment, so be sure to clean immediately after use.

Storage
1. This recipe yields 1–2 servings, so it is intended to be used right away. However, there are no ingredients that will go bad while stored in the refrigerator for a few days. If you do refrigerate this product, you will have to leave it out for a few hours before use because the coconut oil will solidify in the refrigerator.

Directions for Use
1. Rub onto skin in circular motions.
2. Wash off with a warm, damp washcloth. Follow with a cleanser (optional) or an all-natural toner and moisturizer.
3. If it sits on your skin for too long, turmeric may dye your skin orange. Don't worry! This is natural and temporary. If your skin has turned orange, go through your skincare regimen and it should clear up. That being said, it might be best to use turmeric at night before bed, not before a hot date or job interview.

Sensitive Skin Exfoliator

Just because you have sensitive skin doesn't mean you shouldn't exfoliate. Enzymes found in pineapple naturally dissolve dead skins cells, while oats provide gentle exfoliation, perfect for those with sensitive skin.

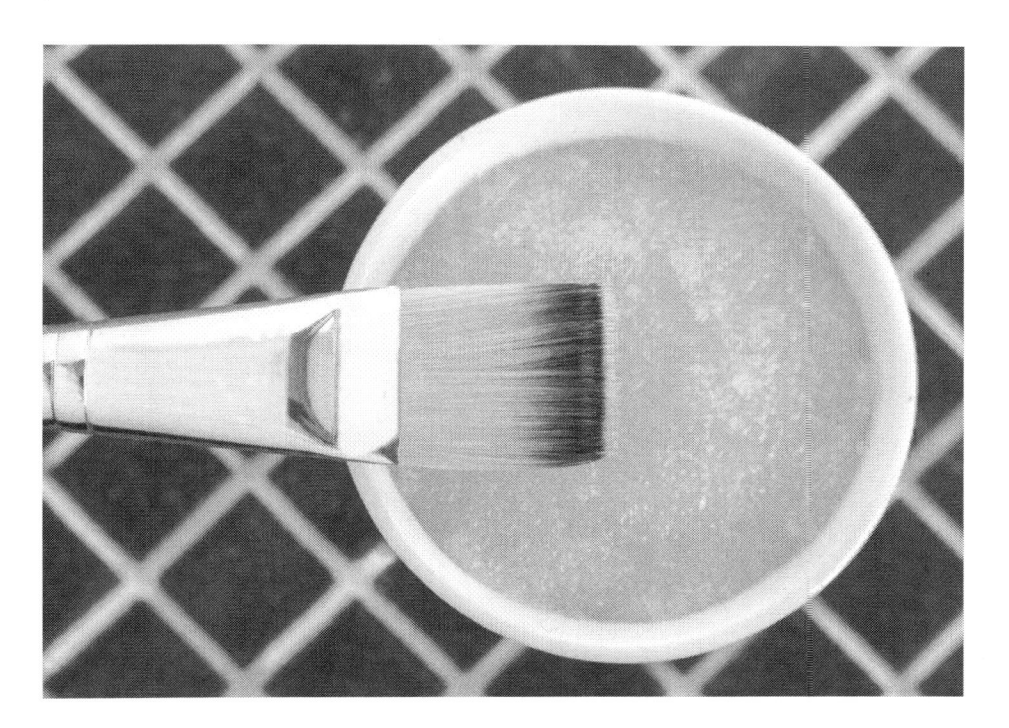

Ingredients

¼ cup pineapple
2 tablespoons rolled oats
2 tablespoons coconut oil

Preparation
1. Combine all ingredients in a blender and blend until smooth. Pour into an airtight container.

Storage
1. Store in the refrigerator in an airtight container for no longer than you would usually store pineapple—no more than one week.

Directions for Use
1. Rub exfoliator onto dry skin in circular motions.
2. Allow to sit on your face for 5 minutes so the pineapple enzymes can do their work.
3. Rinse off with warm water and follow with cleanser (optional) or an all-natural toner and moisturizer.

Mocha Scrub

Coffee wakes up your skin, while cocoa powder delivers a hefty dose of antioxidants. Coffee can also reduce the appearance of cellulite, so feel free to use this scrub on your entire body.

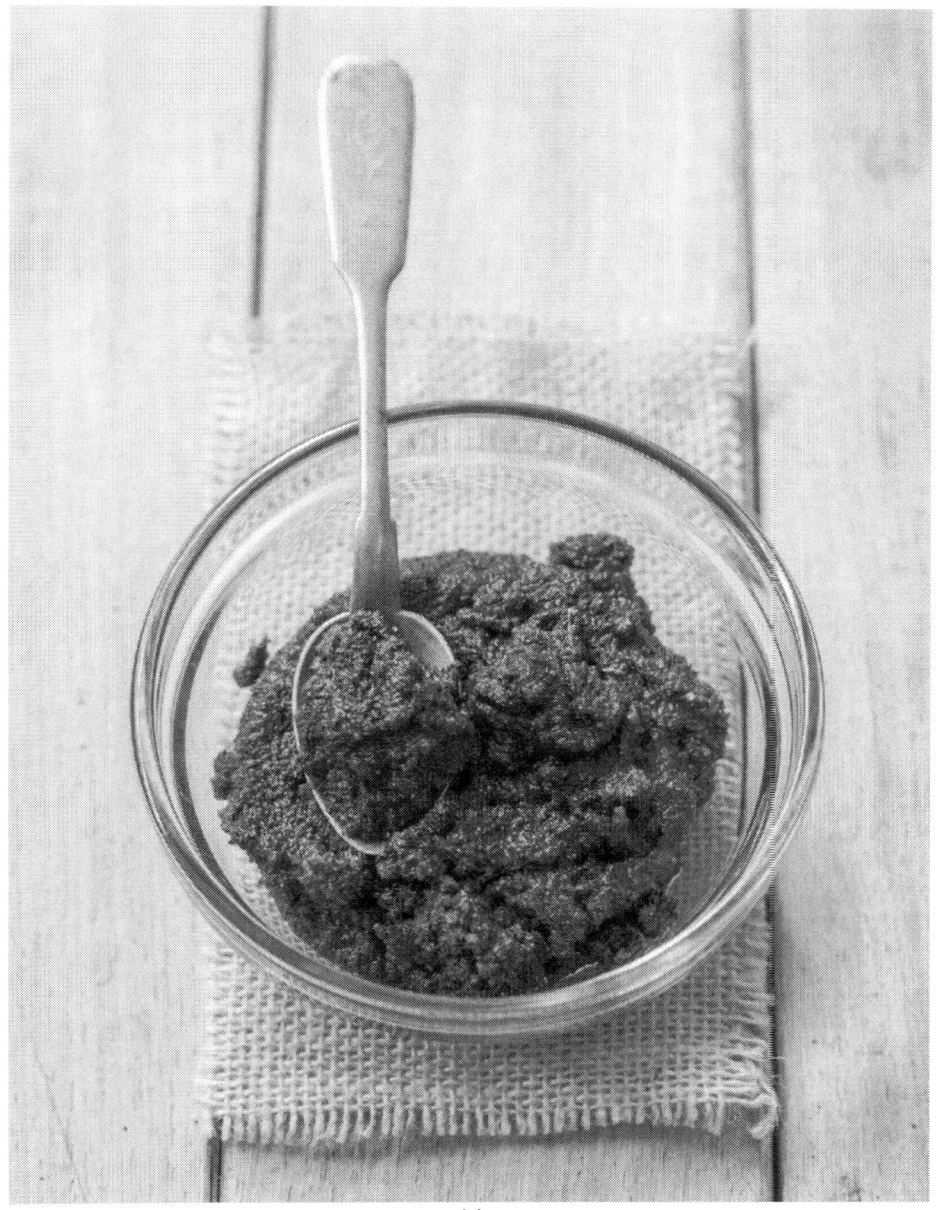

Ingredients

¼ cup coconut oil

2 tablespoons coffee grounds, fresh

2 tablespoons raw cacao powder

Preparation and Directions for Use

1. Combine all ingredients and pour into an airtight container.

Storage

1. Store in an airtight container.

Directions for Use

1. Rub exfoliator onto dry skin in circular motions.
2. Rinse off with warm water and follow with a gentle cleaner and an all-natural toner and moisturizer.

Blackhead Buster

Activated charcoal literally pulls toxins and blackheads out of your pores. Wash your worries down the drain with this powerful but all-natural scrub. This scrub is especially good for body acne, so feel free to use it anywhere.

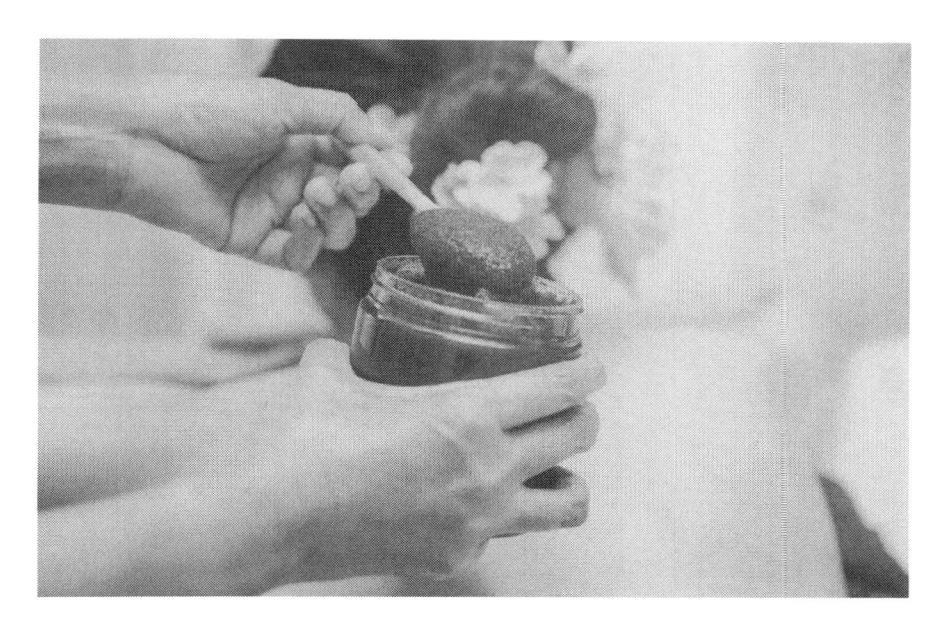

Ingredients
¼ coconut oil
1½ tablespoons activated charcoal
2 drops tea tree essential oil
2 drops lavender essential oil

Preparation
1. Combine all ingredients and pour into an airtight container.

Storage
1. Store in an airtight container.

Directions for Use
1. Rub exfoliator onto dry skin in circular motions.
2. Rinse off with warm water and follow with an all-natural toner and moisturizer.

Rose & Chamomile Exfoliator

Rose and chamomile are both soothing for your skin, so this gentle exfoliator is a great choice for sensitive or aging skin.

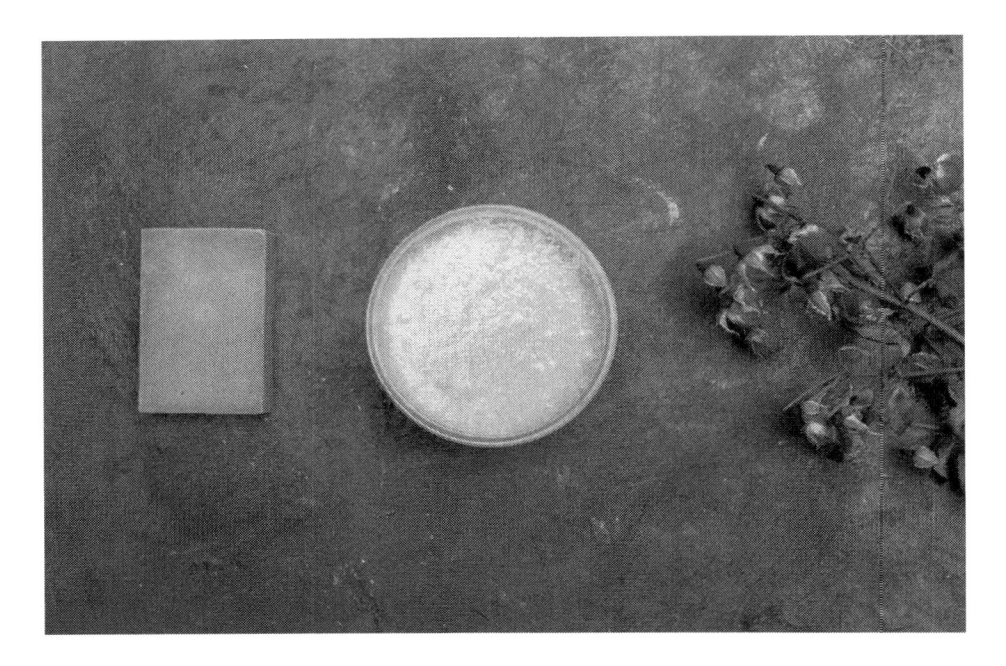

Ingredients
2 tablespoons coconut oil
2 tablespoons rose petal powder
5 drops Roman chamomile essential oil

Preparation
1. Combine all ingredients and pour into an airtight container.

Storage
1. Store in an airtight container in the refrigerator.

Directions for Use
1. Rub exfoliator onto dry skin in circular motions.
2. Rinse off with warm water and follow with an all-natural toner and moisturizer.

Acne Scar Scrub

Fighting acne scars? This scrub might be your best friend. The fruit enzymes in these powerful citrus fruits will dissolve dead skin cells, while lemon oil can lighten acne scars.

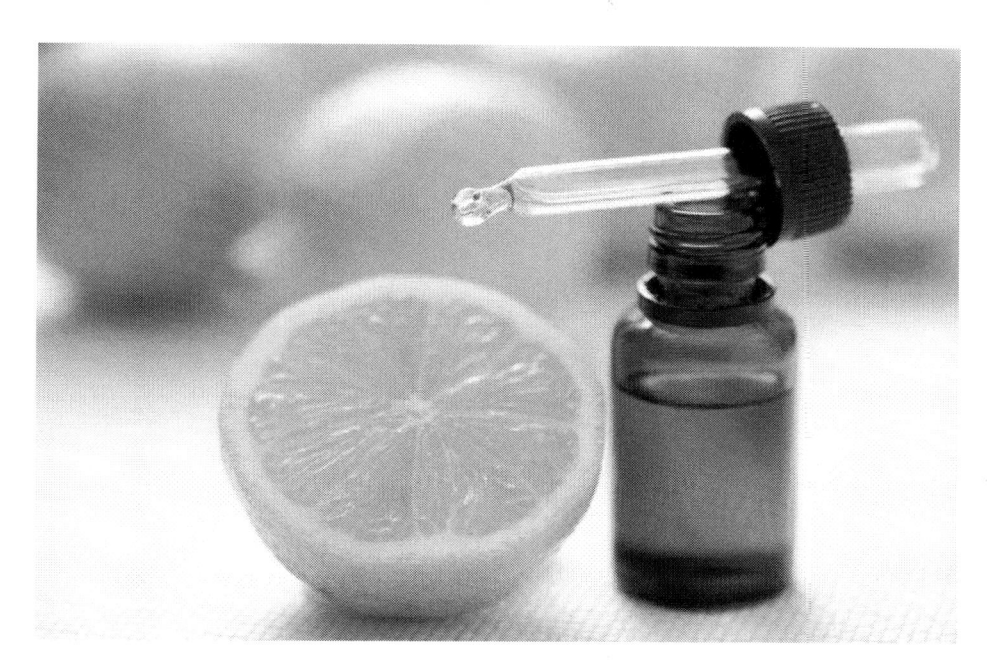

Ingredients
¼ cup coconut oil
10 almonds
1 tablespoon pineapple juice, unsweetened
1 tablespoon orange peel powder
5 drops lemon essential oil

Preparation
1. Blend the almonds and orange peel powder together in a blender or food processor.
2. Once you've made small granules, mix the powder with coconut oil, pineapple juice, and lemon essential oil and pour into an airtight container.

Storage
1. Store in an airtight container in the refrigerator. Only store as long as you would hold onto pineapple juice, about a week.

Directions for Use
1. Rub exfoliator onto dry skin in circular motions.
2. Allow to sit for 5 minutes so fruit enzymes can do their work.
3. Rinse off with warm water and follow with an all-natural toner and moisturizer.

Pink Scrub

Himalayan sea salt is filled with nourishing minerals, 84 to be exact, while providing exfoliation and detoxification to the skin. Meanwhile, grapefruit oil kills bacteria and reduces oil production. If you have oily, acne prone skin, this might be a good choice.

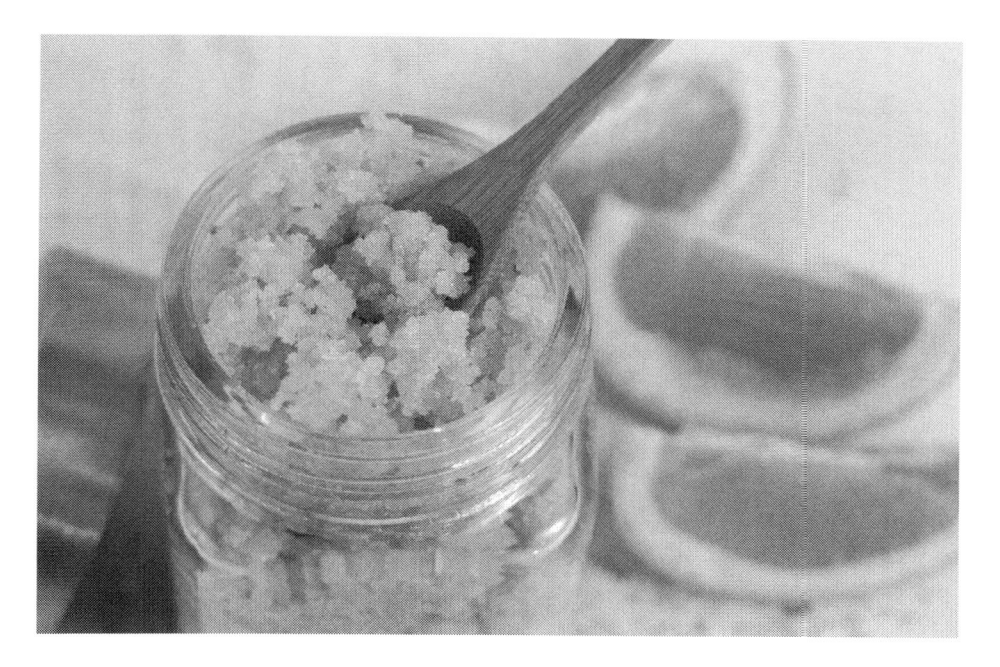

Ingredients
2 tablespoons almond oil
1 tablespoon Himalayan sea salt, finely ground
5 drops pink grapefruit essential oil

Preparation
1. Combine all ingredients and pour into an airtight container.

Storage
1. Store in an airtight container.

Directions for Use
1. Gently rub exfoliator onto dry skin in circular motions.
2. Rinse off with warm water and follow with a gentle cleanser (optional) or an all-natural toner and moisturizer.

Calendula Scrub

Calming calendula combined with moisturizing coconut oil and soothing oats is a gentle exfoliator perfect for aging and sensitive skin.

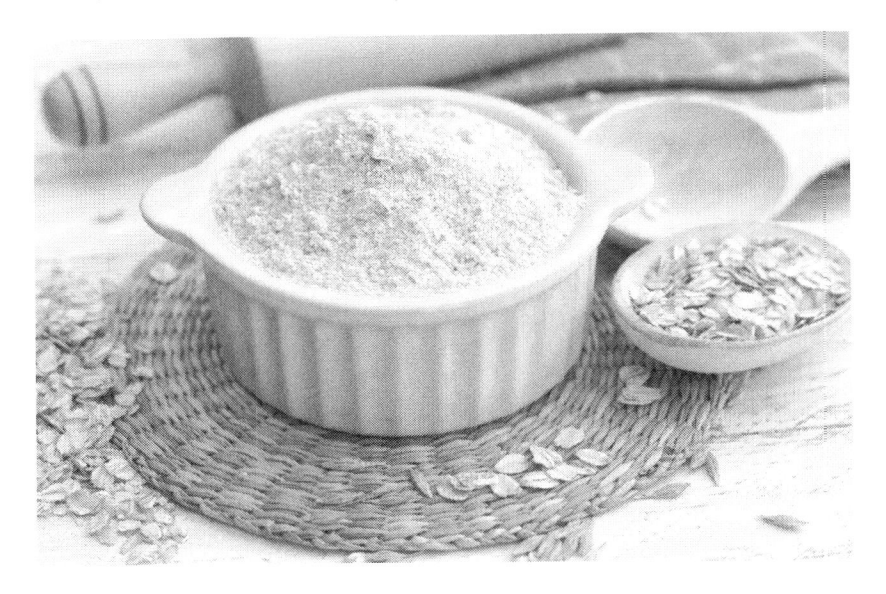

Ingredients
¼ cup coconut oil
2 tablespoons calendula powder
2 tablespoons rolled oats
5 drops lavender essential oil

Preparation
1. Grind the rolled oats in a blender or food processor until you have a fine powder.
2. Mix together with the calendula powder and oil and pour into an airtight container.

Storage
1. Store in an airtight container in the refrigerator.

Directions for Use
1. Rub exfoliator onto dry skin in circular motions.
2. Rinse off with warm water and follow with an all-natural toner and moisturizer.

Toners

Rosewater Toner

Rosewater is a moisturizing treat for your skin—plus, it covers up the smell of apple cider vinegar (ACV). Together they smooth the skin and work wonders for acne, while leaving you smelling wonderful.

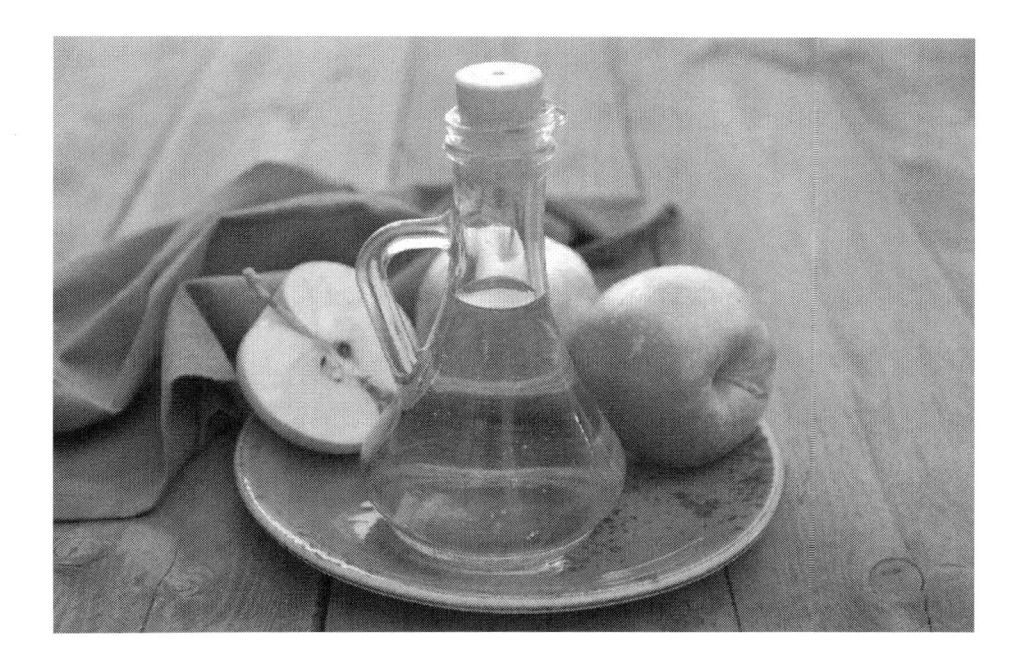

Ingredients
1 cup rosewater
2 tablespoons ACV

Preparation
1. Mix ingredients together and pour into an airtight container.

Storage
1. Store in an airtight container in the refrigerator.

Directions for Use
1. Shake well before use.
2. Pour about a quarter-sized amount of toner onto a cotton pad and rub all over your face, neck, chest, and back. Use more if needed.
3. Follow with an all-natural moisturizer.

Goodnight Toner

Chamomile tea mixed with lavender and cedarwood is the perfect combination to put you to sleep. It's also a soothing blend for sensitive skin, while the anti-inflammatory agents will help to soothe skin irritation and cystic acne.

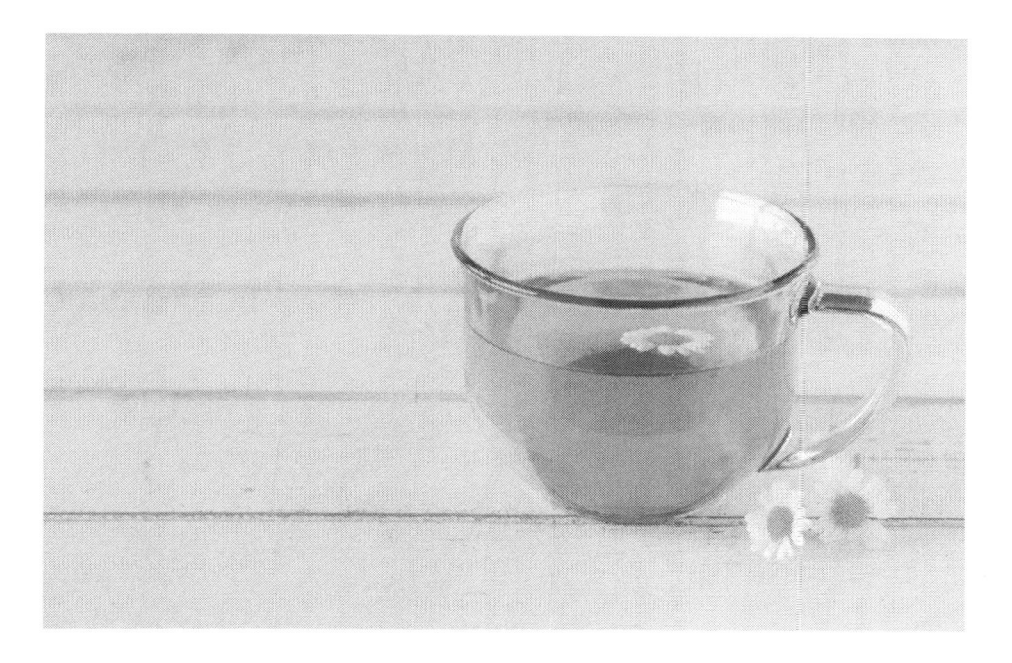

Ingredients
1 cup chamomile tea
2 tablespoons ACV
7 drops lavender essential oil
4 drops cedarwood essential oil

Preparation
1. Mix ingredients together and pour into an airtight container.

Storage
1. Store in an airtight container in the refrigerator.

Directions for Use
1. Shake well before use.
2. Pour about a quarter-sized amount of toner onto a cotton pad and rub all over your face, neck, chest, and back. Use more if needed.
3. Follow with an all-natural moisturizer.

Antioxidant Toner

This toner features free-radical-scavenging green tea combined with some of the essential oils highest in antioxidants. Plus, blue tansy, lavender, and geranium are all said to have a calming effect on the mind.

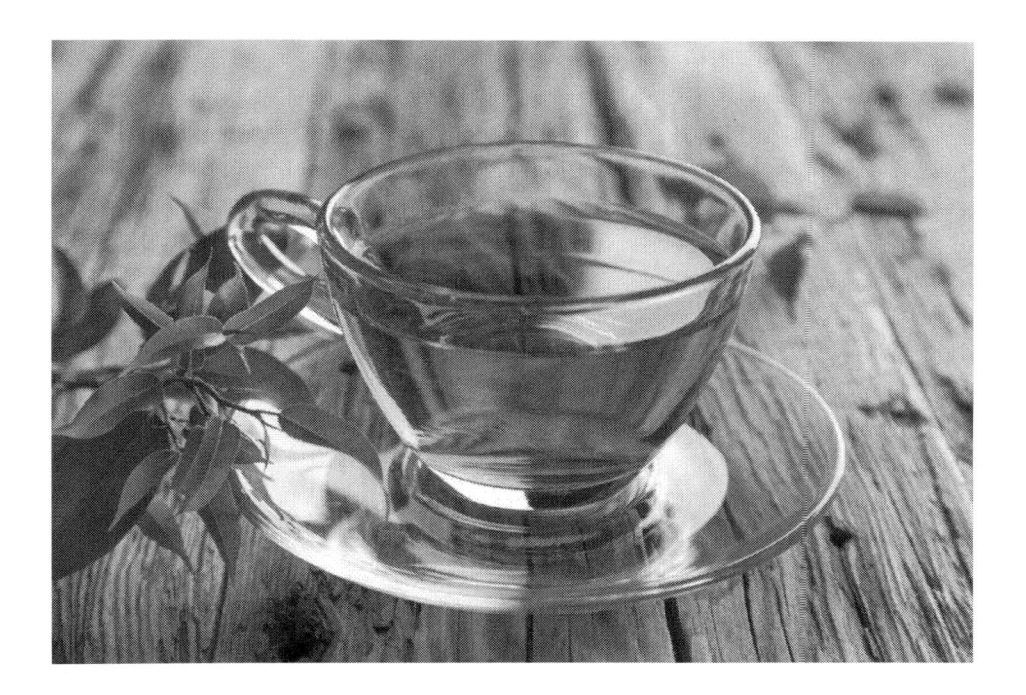

Ingredients

1 cup green tea
2 tablespoons ACV
5 drops blue tansy essential oil
3 drops geranium essential oil
2 drops lavender essential oil

Preparation
1. Mix ingredients together and pour into an airtight container.

Storage
1. Store in the refrigerator in an airtight container.

Directions for Use
1. Shake well before use.
2. Pour about a quarter-sized amount of toner onto a cotton pad and rub all over your face, neck, chest, and back. Use more if needed.
3. Follow with an all-natural moisturizer.

Aloe Toner

Aloe vera juice is healing, with anti-inflammatory properties, while witch hazel works as an astringent and tea tree oil treats blemishes. Coconut water adds an antimicrobial element. Together, these ingredients make for a healing acne treatment that's especially good for cystic acne and inflammation. Wanna go the extra mile? Grow your own aloe vera plants and squeeze out the juice yourself.

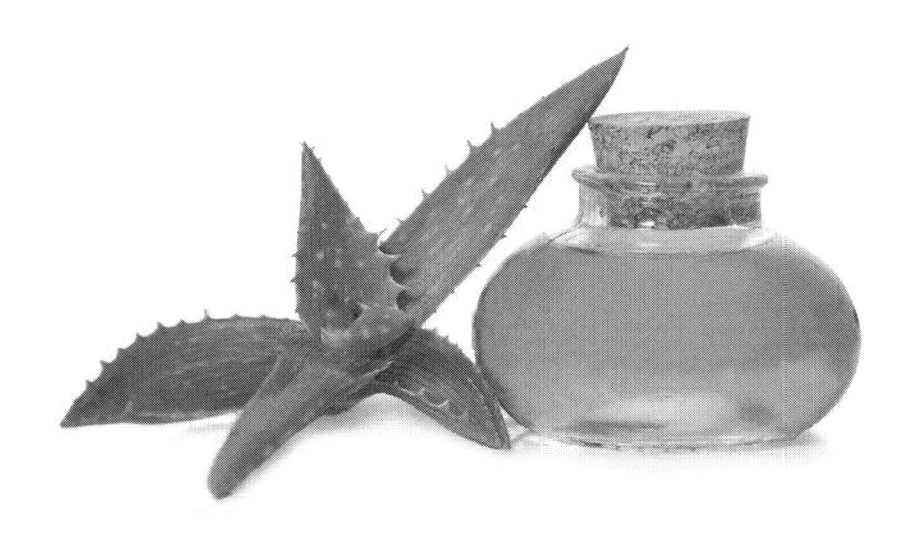

Ingredients
¼ cup aloe vera juice
½ cup coconut water
2 tablespoons witch hazel
5 drops tea tree oil

Preparation
1. Mix ingredients together and pour into an airtight container.

Storage
1. Store in the refrigerator in an airtight container.

Directions for Use
1. Shake well before use.
2. Pour about a quarter-sized amount of toner onto a cotton pad and rub all over your face, neck, chest, and back. Use more if needed.
3. Follow with an all-natural moisturizer.

Elderberry Toner

Elderberry and green tea are powerful antioxidants, while the lauric acid in coconut provides an additional anti-aging effect. This toner is also ultra-soothing, perfect for sensitive skin.

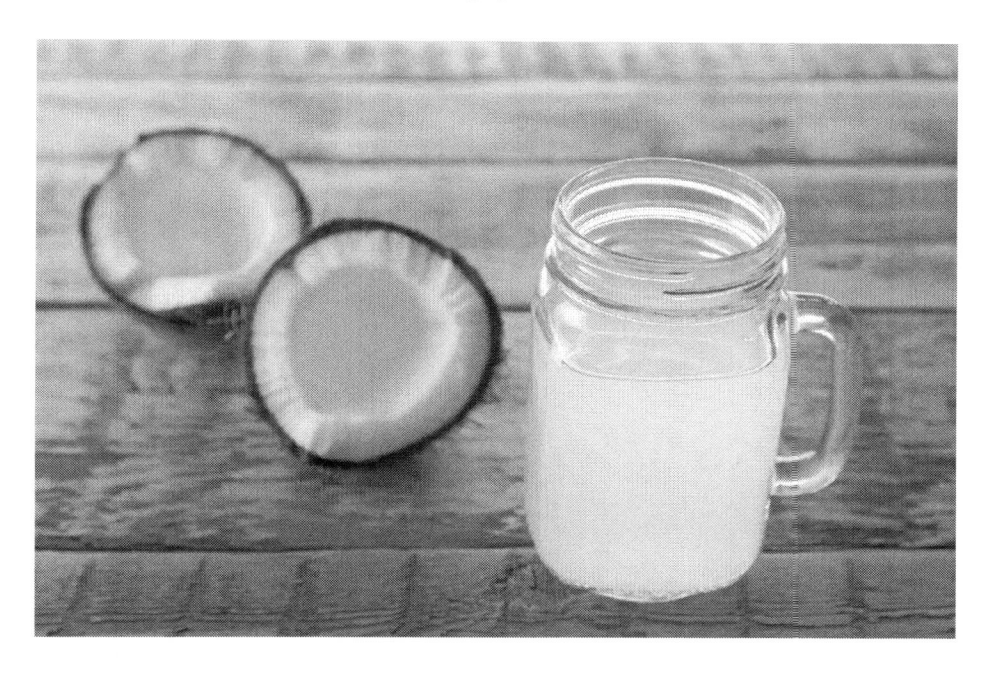

Ingredients
½ cup green tea
½ cup coconut water
10 drops elderberry extract

Preparation
1. Mix ingredients together and pour into an airtight container.

Storage
1. Store in the refrigerator in an airtight container.

Directions for Use
1. Shake well before use.
2. Pour about a quarter-sized amount of toner onto a cotton pad and rub all over your face, neck, chest, and back. Use more if needed.
3. Follow with an all-natural moisturizer.

Acne Toner

Willow bark contains the acne-fighting ingredient salicylic acid, in an all-natural form, and also has an anti-inflammatory effect. Add this to your regimen if you're fighting acne, especially cystic acne.

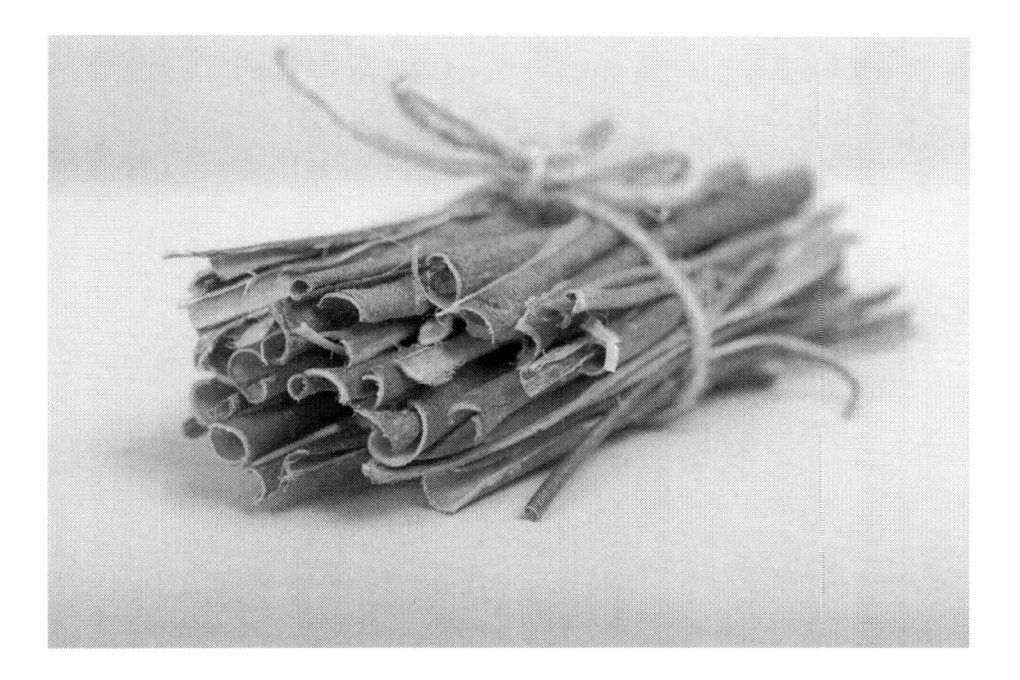

Ingredients
1 cup water
2 tablespoons witch hazel
1 tablespoon white willow bark
5 drops tea tree essential oil
5 drops lavender essential oil

Preparation
1. Bring 1 cup of water to a boil. In a coffee filter or tea infuser, add the willow bark to the hot water.
2. Soak for 10 minutes, then remove the willow bark.

3. Mix the apple cider vinegar into the tea and add the essential oils.
4. Pour into an airtight container.

Storage
1. Store in the refrigerator in an airtight container.

Directions for Use
1. Shake well before use.
2. Pour about a quarter-sized amount of toner onto a cotton pad and rub all over your face, neck, chest, and back. Use more if needed.
3. Follow with an all-natural moisturizer.

Lavender Lemonade

Thought lavender lemonade was just a delicious summer beverage? Wrong! Lavender soothes skin, while lemon lightens scars and hyperpigmentation. This toner smells so good you'll want to drink it. Like most of the recipes in this book, you technically can!

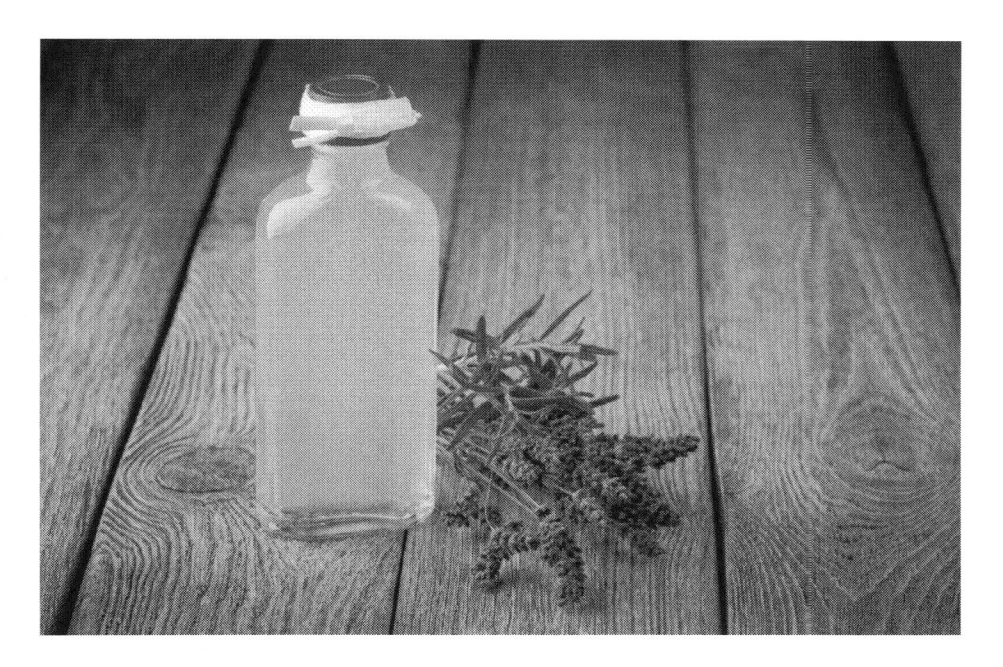

Ingredients
1 cup coconut water
2 tablespoons ACV
5 drops lavender essential oil
5 drops lemon essential oil

Preparation
1. Mix ingredients together and pour into an airtight container.

Storage
1. Store in the refrigerator in an airtight container.

Directions for Use
1. Shake well before use.
2. Pour about a quarter-sized amount of toner onto a cotton pad and rub all over your face, neck, chest, and back. Use more if needed.
3. Follow with an all-natural moisturizer.

Rosemary Rice Toner

Rice water is said to help achieve glowing skin, while antiseptic rosemary is great for acne and preventing sun damage, making this toner a good choice for virtually any skin type.

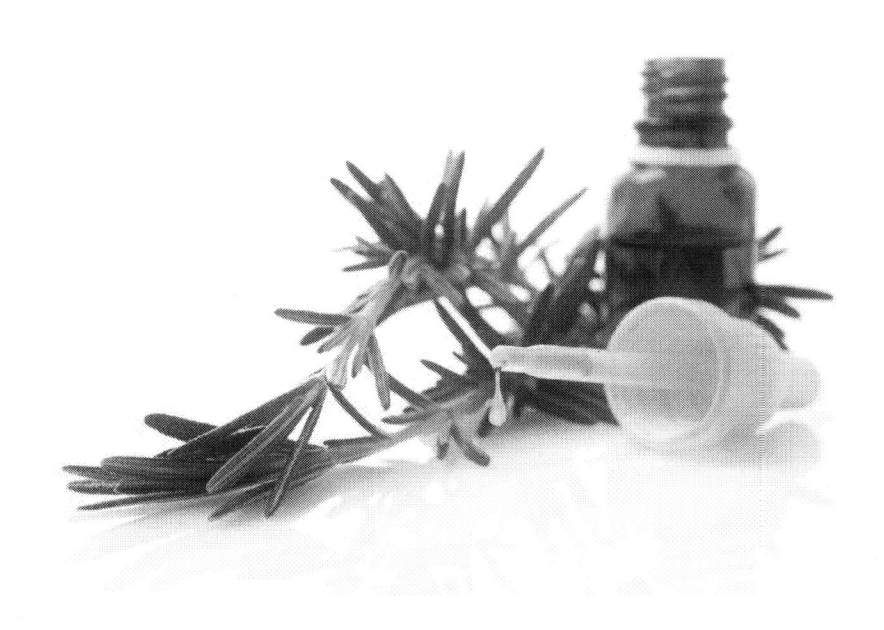

Ingredients
1¼ cups water
½ cup rice
10 drops rosemary essential oil
2 drops lavender essential oil

Preparation
1. In a large bowl, soak the rice in the water for about 15 minutes.
2. Once the water is milky, strain out the rice.
3. Mix the water with the essential oils and pour into an airtight container.

Storage
1. Store in the refrigerator in an airtight container.

Directions for Use
1. Shake well before use.
2. Pour about a quarter-sized amount of toner onto a cotton pad and rub all over your face, neck, chest, and back. Use more if needed.
3. Follow with an all-natural moisturizer.

Moisturizers

Aloe Butter

Cocoa butter and aloe gel together are a super healing combination. Put this on wounds, burns, sunburns, and scars, or use at night and wake up to new skin.

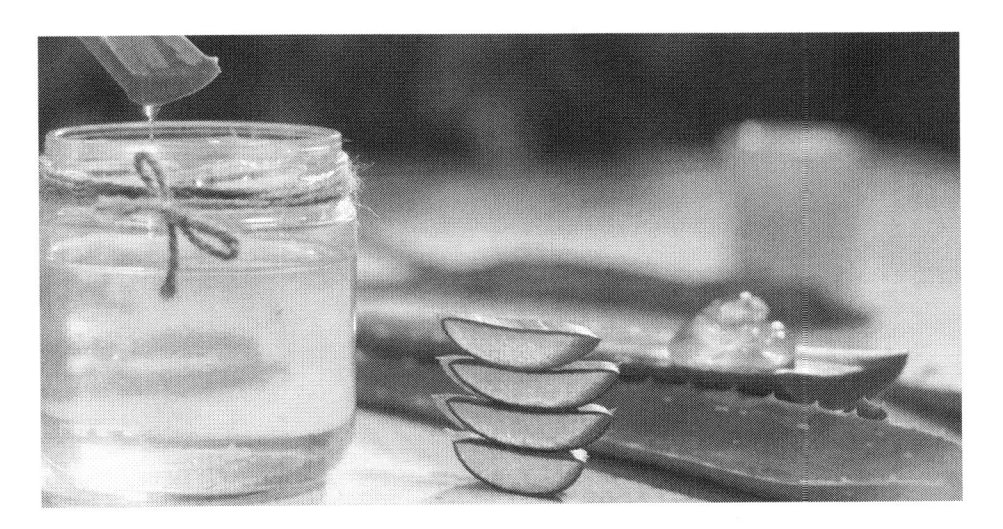

Ingredients

½ cup cocoa butter
2 tablespoons mango butter
2 tablespoons aloe vera gel
6 drops lavender essential oil
3 drops rosemary essential oil

Preparation

1. Melt the cocoa butter slightly and mix together the other ingredients. Scoop into an airtight container.

Storage
1. Store in an airtight container in the refrigerator for up to a month.

Directions for Use
1. Begin by rubbing a dime-sized amount into the desired area. Use more if needed depending on how dry your skin is or how severe the burn.

Eczema Cream

Itchy eczema is not only uncomfortable, it can also be unsightly. This super-soothing cream should help.

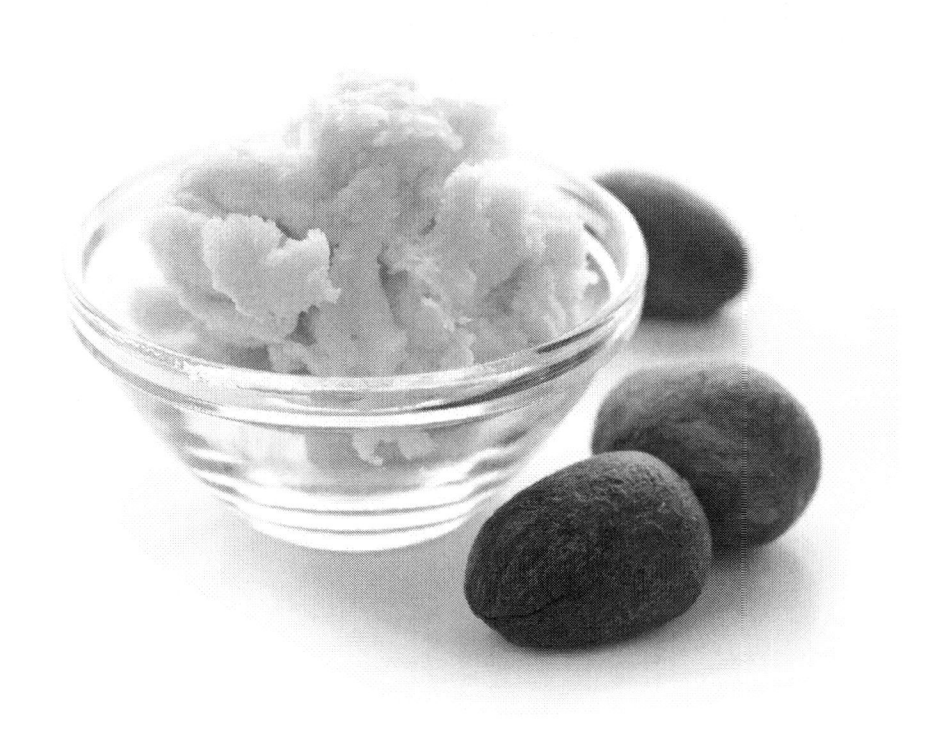

Ingredients
½ cup shea butter
¼ cup coconut oil
2 tablespoons rolled oats, ground
15 drops lavender essential oil
5 drops tea tree essential oil
5 drops Roman chamomile essential oil

Preparations
1. Finely grind the oats in a food processor, blender, or coffee grinder.
2. Melt the shea butter slightly and mix together with the other ingredients. It should not be so hot that it cooks the oats, only warm enough to mix well.
3. Scoop into an airtight container.

Storage
1. Store in an airtight container in the refrigerator.

Directions for Use
1. Begin by rubbing a dime-sized amount into the desired area. Use more if needed depending on how severe the eczema is.

Blue Moisturizer

Looking for a super-hydrating moisturizer loaded with antioxidants? Look no further, anti-inflammatory and detoxifying blue spirulina is the antioxidant mother lode.

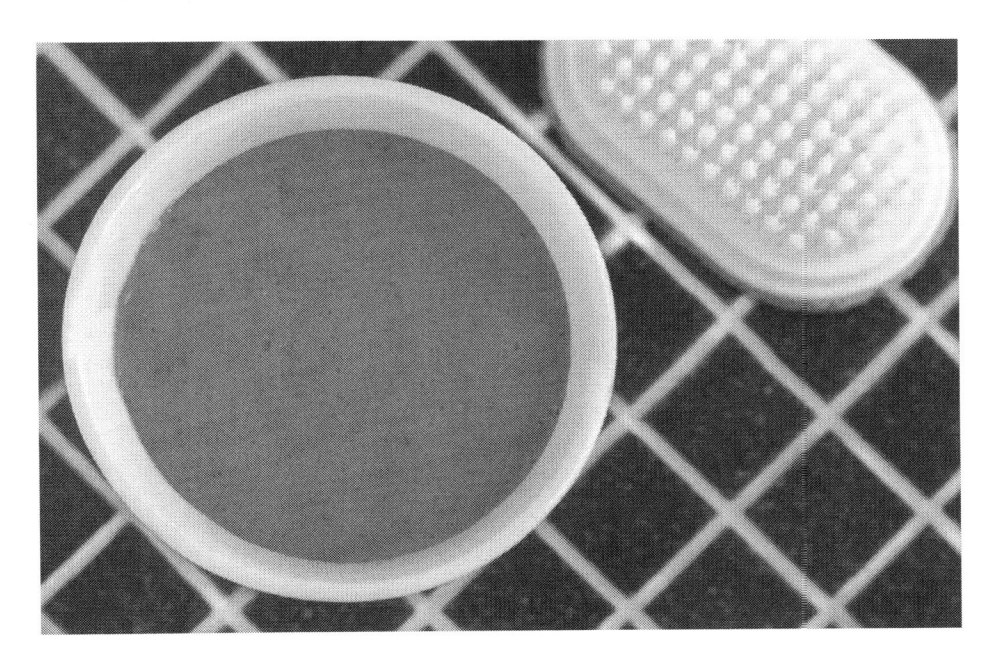

Ingredients
½ cup sweet almond oil
½ cup shea butter
1 teaspoon blue spirulina
10 drops blue tansy essential oil

Preparation
1. Melt the shea butter slightly and mix together with the sweet almond oil.
2. Add spirulina and blue tansy oil once the mixture has cooled slightly.
3. Scoop into an airtight container in the refrigerator.

Storage
1. Store in an airtight container.

Directions for Use
1. Begin by rubbing a dime-sized amount into the desired area. Use more if needed depending on how dry your skin is.

Lemon Butter

This moisturizer is citrusy and oh so refreshing. Plus, lemon is brightening and can help reduce the appearance of acne scars.

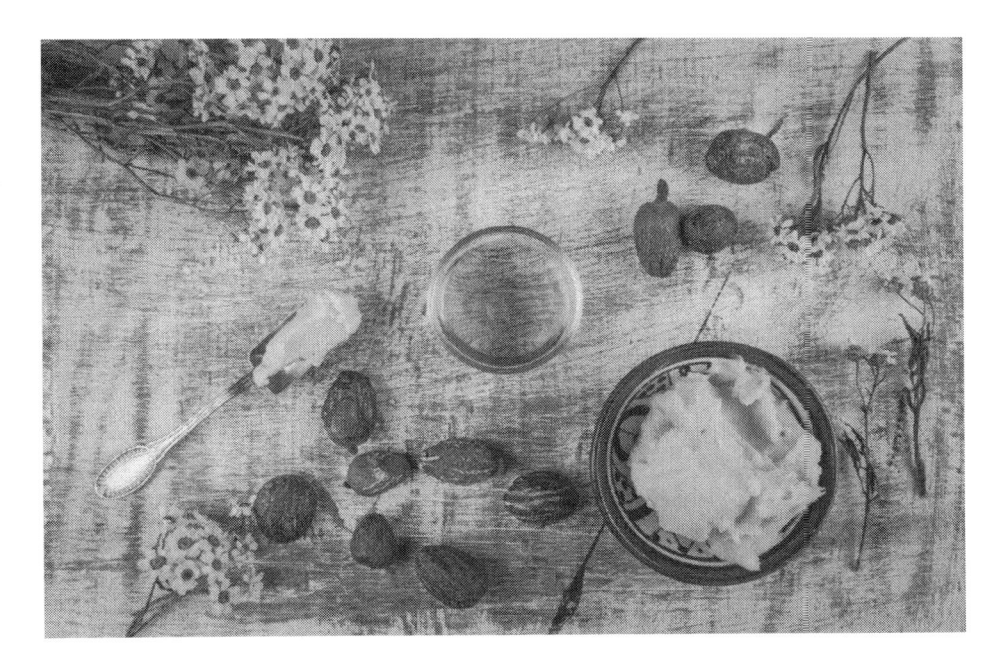

Ingredients
½ cup shea butter
2 tablespoons jojoba oil
10 drops lemon essential oil

Preparation
1. Melt the shea butter slightly and mix together the other ingredients.
2. Scoop into an airtight container.

Storage
1. Store in an airtight container.

Directions for Use
1. Begin by rubbing a dime-sized amount into the desired area. Use more if needed depending on how dry your skin is.

Brightening Serum

This serum is a heavy-duty moisturizer perfect for just before bed. These powerful essential oils will have you looking radiant in no time and will also decrease the appearance of acne scars.

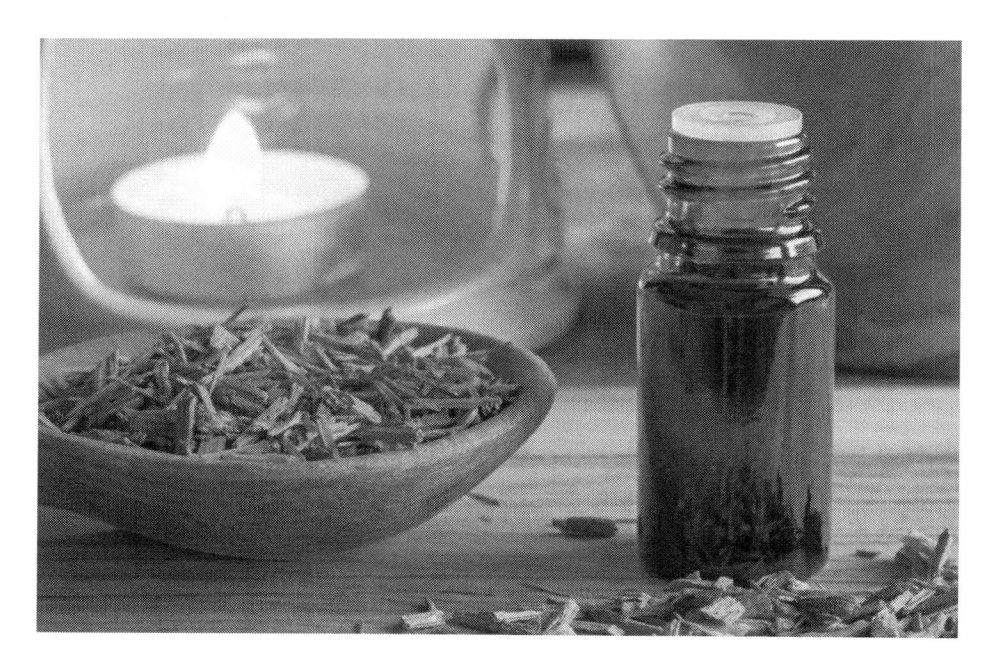

Ingredients
¼ cup jojoba oil
5 drops sandalwood essential oil
5 drops carrot seed oil
3 drops blue tansy essential oil
2 drops lemongrass essential oil

Preparation
1. Mix all ingredients together and scoop into an airtight container.

Storage
1. Store in an airtight container.

Directions for Use
1. Begin by rubbing a dime-sized amount into the desired area. Use more if needed depending on how dry your skin is.

Frankincense and Myrrh

Prized in ancient times, the sensual smell of frankincense and myrrh is still the height of luxury. This skincare duo wasn't just used as a gift for kings; it was also used on skin in ancient Egypt. Myrrh was even used in mummification! Today, frankincense and myrrh still smell amazing, and they're also used as a powerful anti-aging combo.

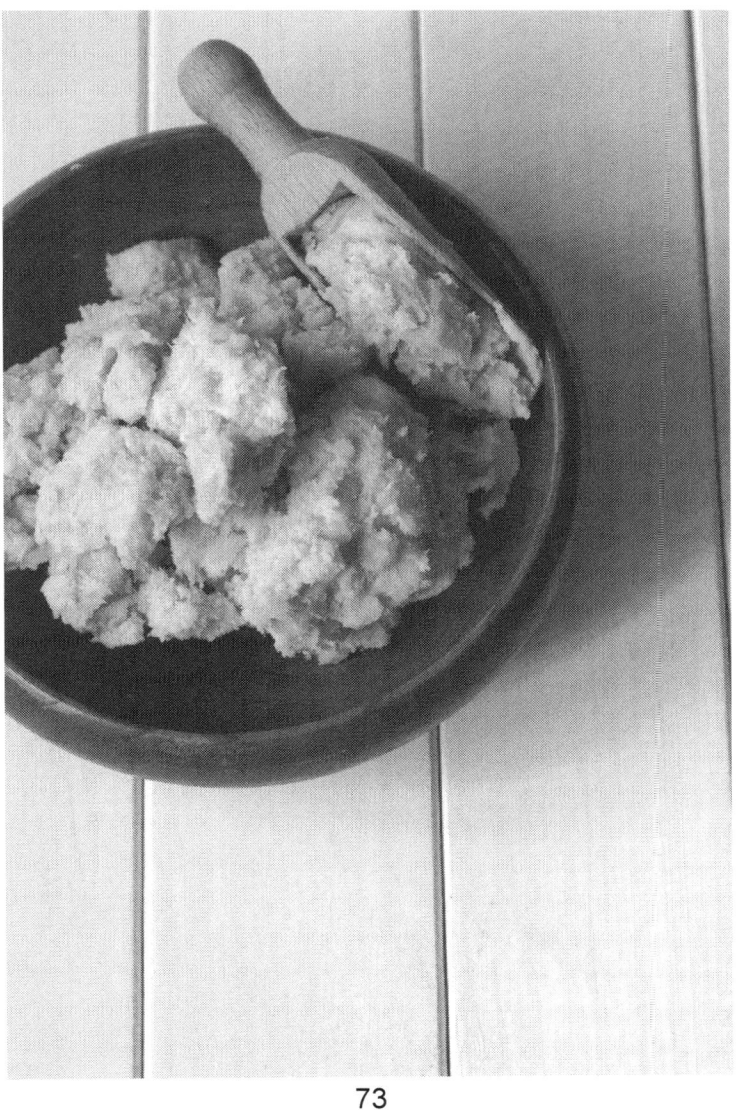

Ingredients

½ cup shea butter
2 tablespoons argan oil
5 drops frankincense essential oil
5 drops myrrh essential oil

Preparation

1. Melt the shea butter slightly and mix together with the other ingredients.
2. Scoop into an airtight container.

Storage

1. Store in an airtight container.

Directions for Use

1. Begin by rubbing a dime-sized amount into the desired area. Use more if needed depending on how dry your skin is.

Anti-Aging Eye Cream

The delicate skin around your eyes is often where the first signs of aging show up. Give your skin the care it needs to prevent premature aging with this antioxidant-rich eye cream.

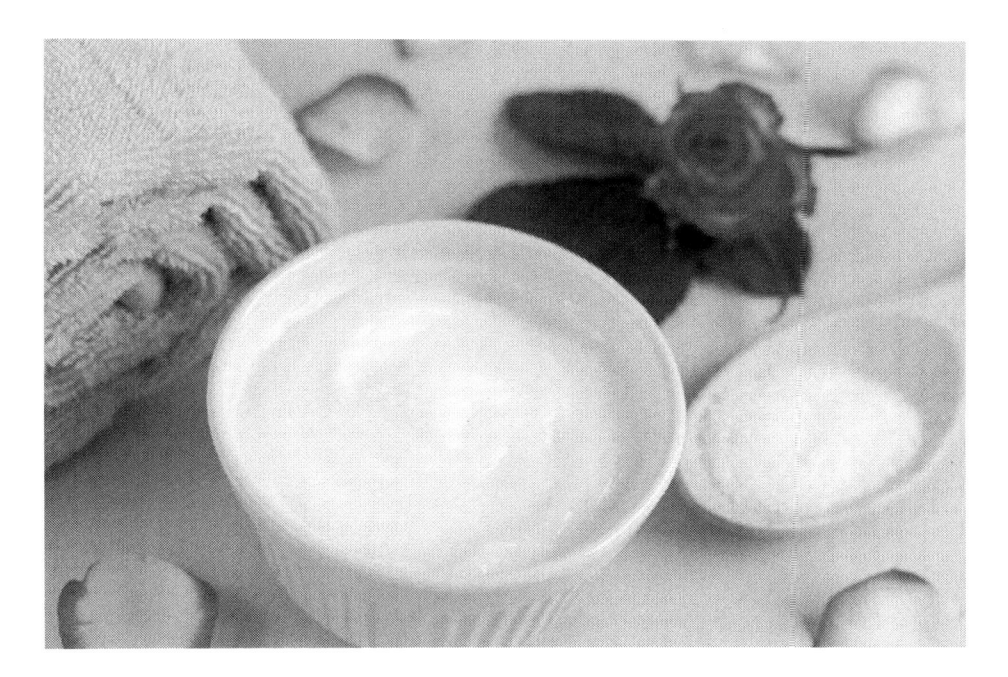

Ingredients
¼ cup shea butter
2 tablespoons argan oil
5 drops rose hip oil
5 drops carrot seed oil
2 drops pomegranate seed oil
2 drops geranium essential oil

Preparation
1. Melt the shea butter slightly and mix together the other ingredients. Do not mix if the shea butter is hot; wait until it has cooled slightly.
2. Scoop into an airtight container.

Storage
1. Store in an airtight container.

Directions for Use
1. Begin by rubbing a dime-sized amount into the desired area. Use more if needed depending on how dry your skin is.

Acne Prone Moisturizer

If you have oily, acne prone skin you may hesitate to moisturize, but not moisturizing actually causes your skin to overproduce oil to compensate, only leading to more acne in the long run. Try this instead. Tea tree oil and rosemary are astringents that treat acne, while jojoba oil provides a lovely moisturizing effect.

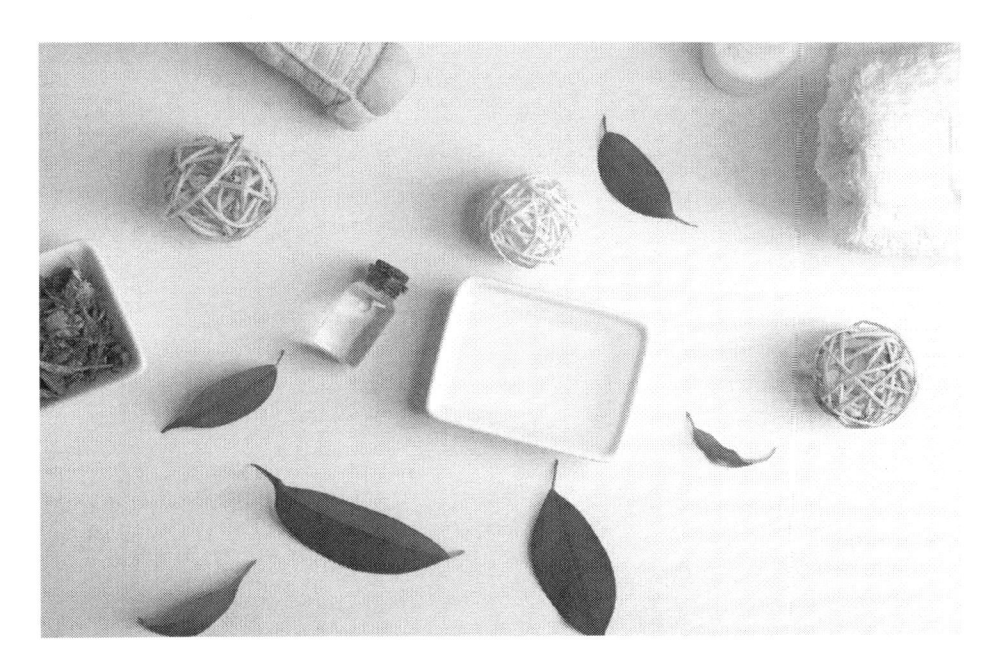

Ingredients
¼ cup jojoba oil
2 tablespoons shea butter
5 drops rosemary essential oil
3 drops tea tree essential oil

Preparation
1. Melt the shea butter slightly and mix together with the other ingredients.
2. Scoop into an airtight container.

Storage
1. Store in an airtight container.

Directions for Use
1. Begin by rubbing a dime-sized amount into the desired area. Use more if needed depending on how dry your skin is.

Masks

Rose Mask

Rose clay is not only beautiful, it's also a gentle exfoliator and detoxifier perfect for sensitive skin. Combine with rose hip seed oil and apple cider vinegar and you've got yourself a powerful cleansing mask. Great for mature skin, too!

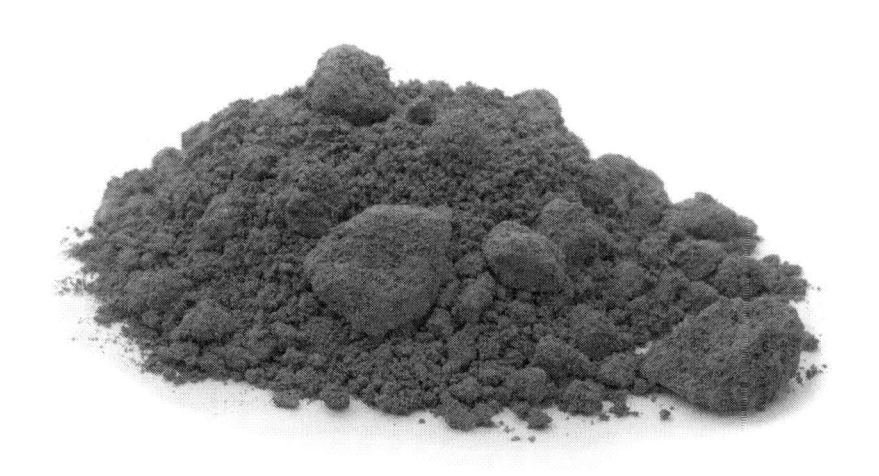

Ingredients
2 tablespoons ACV
1 tablespoon rose clay
5 drops rose hip seed oil

Preparation
1. Mix together until smooth. Use immediately as the clay will dry out.

Storage
1. This recipe only makes enough for one use because the clay will dry out. No need to store, just use right away!

Directions for Use
1. Rub onto dry, clean skin.
2. Wait 10–15 minutes until the clay is dry, then rinse off with warm water. Follow with an all-natural toner or moisturizer, or your entire normal skincare routine.

Papaya Mask

Papaya has naturally occurring enzymes that dissolve dead skins cells and brighten skin. This mask is a good choice for those with sensitive skin who still want to exfoliate.

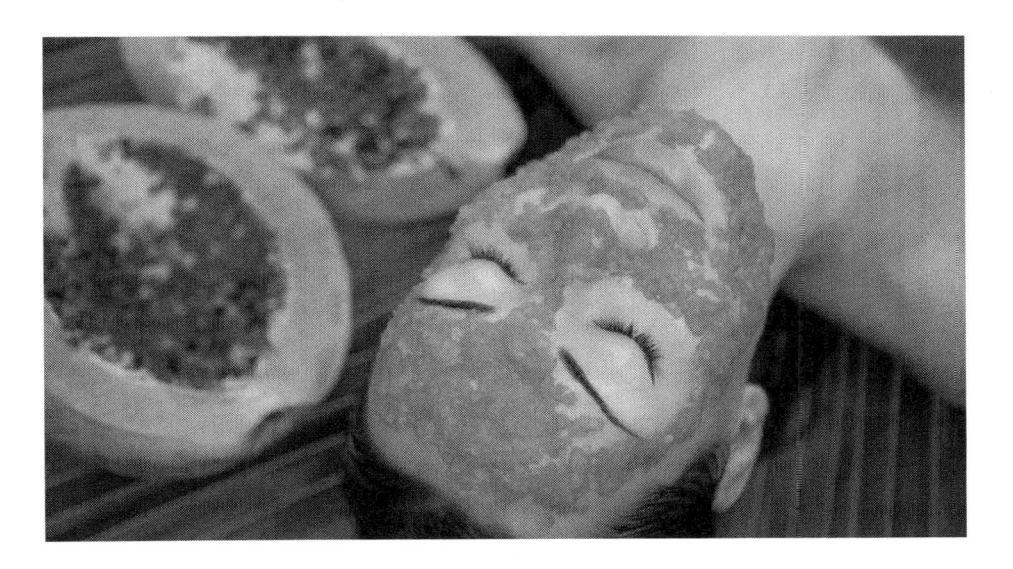

Ingredients
¼ cup papaya, peeled and cubed
2 tablespoons mango butter

Preparation
1. Combine ingredients in the blender. Blend until smooth. Scoop into an airtight container.

Storage
1. Store in an airtight container in the refrigerator. Do not store longer than you would normally hold onto papaya—no more than one week.

Directions for Use

1. Smooth over face and allow to sit for 10–15 minutes so papaya enzymes can work their magic.
2. Wash off in circular motions.
3. This mask should leave your face feeling moisturized, but feel free to follow with an all-natural toner and moisturizer. You can also carry on with your normal skincare routine if you'd like.

Bentonite Mask

Bentonite clay is incredibly detoxifying, so you should use this mask on your whole body. The clay has a suction effect, so you may feel a tingling sensation and your skin might be red for about 30 minutes after use. Because it can leave your skin looking red and blotchy, it's recommended that you use this mask before bed, not in the morning before work.

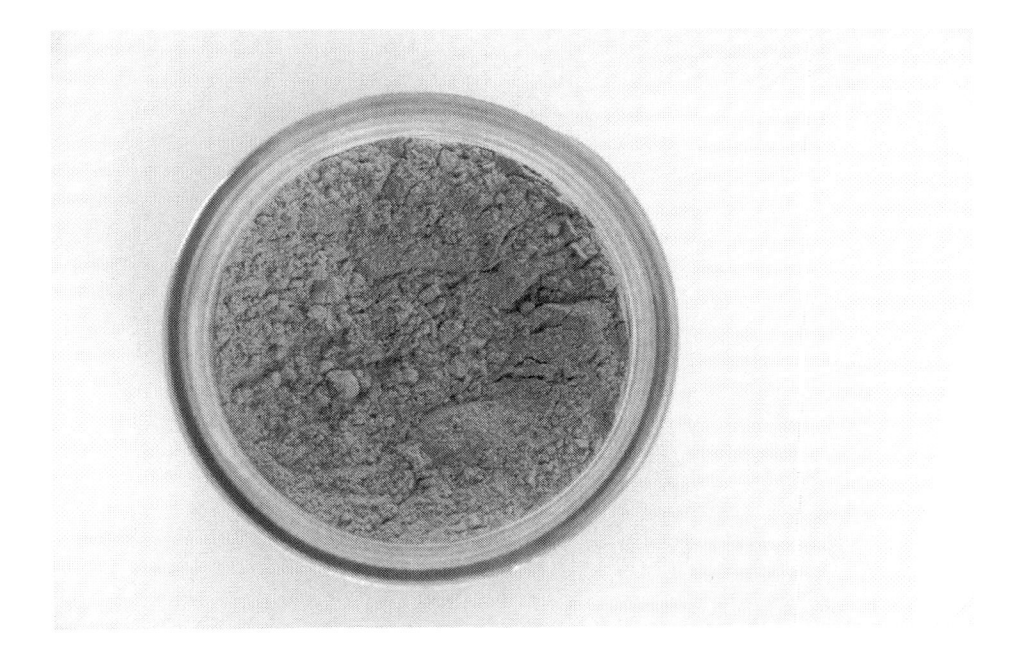

Ingredients
2 tablespoons bentonite clay
1 tablespoon rose powder
3 drops lavender essential oil
ACV (as needed)

Preparation
1. Combine all ingredients, adding apple cider vinegar as needed until you have a smooth paste.
2. Use immediately.

Storage
1. This recipe only makes enough for 1–2 uses, because the clay will dry out if you try to store it.
2. If you have any of the mask left over, use it on your body. It's especially nice on the bottom of your feet.

Directions for Use
1. Rub onto dry, clean skin in a thick layer.
2. Wait 10–15 minutes until the clay is dry, then rinse off with warm water. Follow with an all-natural toner or moisturizer, or your entire normal skincare routine.

Turmeric Mask

Turmeric is an incredibly powerful way to brighten and firm skin, so a little goes a long way! It's also great for acne and comes loaded with powerful antioxidants.

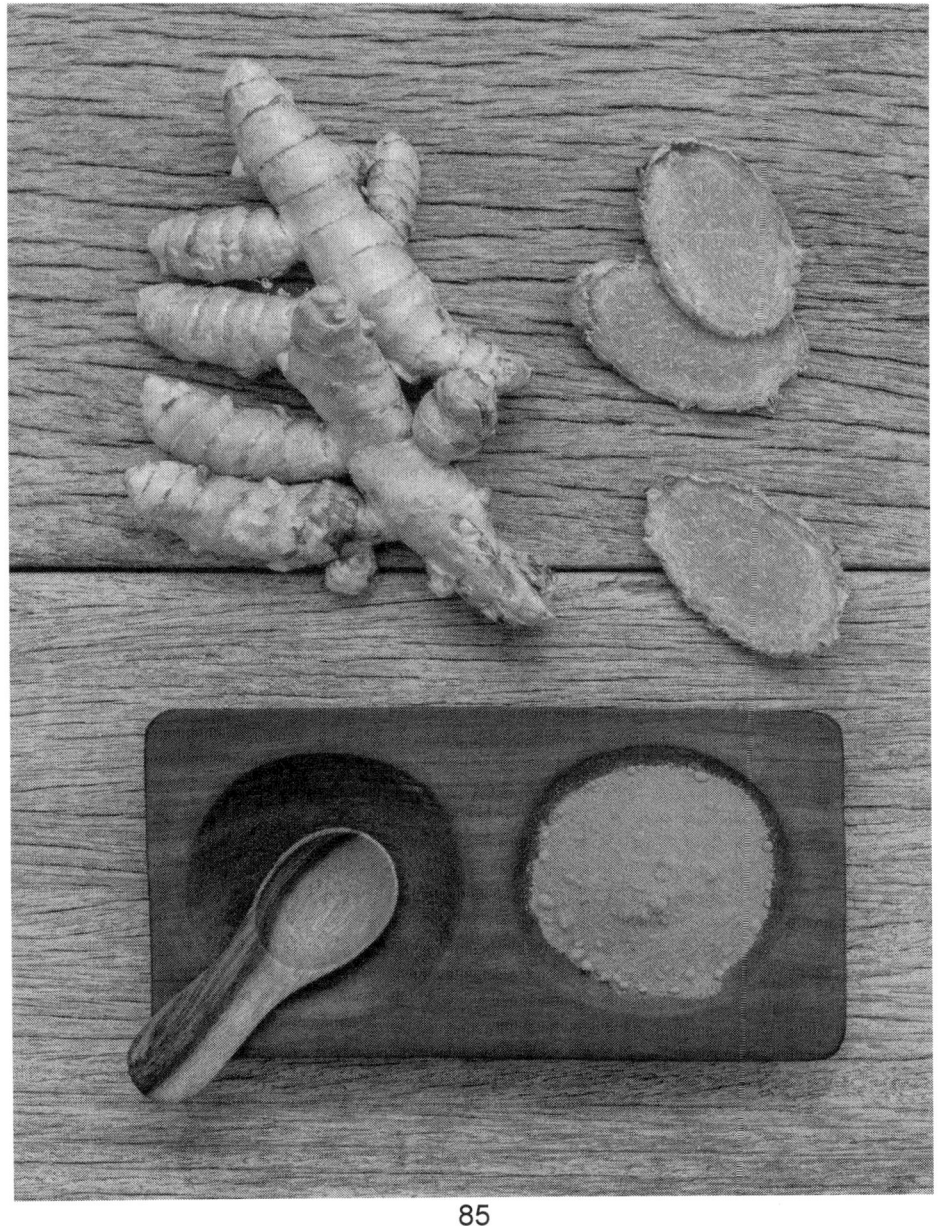

Ingredients

1 teaspoon turmeric
1 teaspoon almond milk
3 drops sandalwood essential oil
ACV (as needed)

Preparation

1. Combine all ingredients, adding apple cider vinegar as needed until you have a smooth paste.
2. Use immediately.

Storage

1. This recipe only makes enough for 1–2 uses, because turmeric might dry out if you try to store it.
2. If you have any of the mask left over, use it on your body. It's especially nice on the bottom of your feet.

Directions for Use

1. Rub onto dry, clean skin in an even layer.
2. Wait 10–15 minutes until the turmeric is dry, then remove with a warm, damp washcloth. Follow with an all-natural toner or moisturizer, or your entire normal skincare routine.
3. Turmeric may dye your skin orange, so this is best to use at night. If your skin does look orange, don't scrub it roughly, because this could cause irritation. Just carry on with your normal skincare routine.

Banana and Oats Mask

This mask is incredibly soothing for irritated, dry, or sensitive skin. Banana comes loaded with vitamins C and E, while oats soothe and moisturize the skin. Plus, it's good enough to eat!

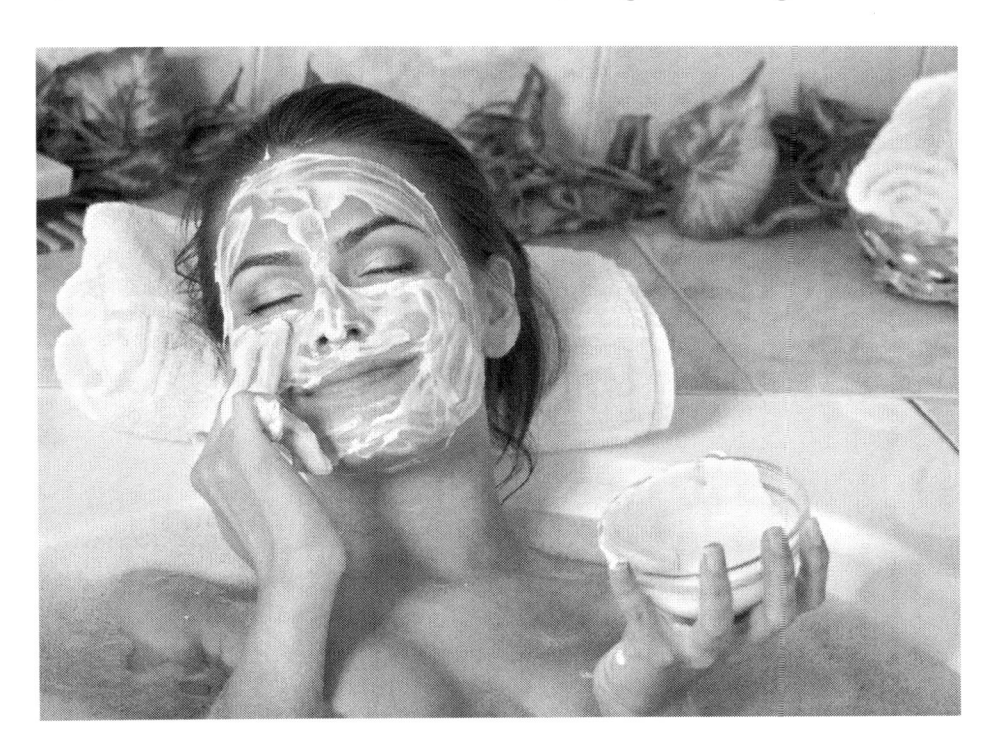

Ingredients
¼ banana
3 tablespoons rolled oats
1 teaspoon almond milk

Preparation
1. Blend ingredients together in the blender.
2. Scoop into an airtight container.

Storage
1. Store in an airtight container in the refrigerator. Do not store longer than you would normally hold onto banana in the refrigerator—no more than one week.

Directions for Use
1. Smooth over face and allow to sit for 10–15 minutes.
2. Wash off in circular motions.
3. This mask should leave your face feeling moisturized, but feel free to follow with an all-natural toner and moisturizer. You can also carry on with your normal skincare routine if you'd like.

Flaxseed Mask

Because you're a vegan, you probably choose not to use an egg white face mask. This mask provides similar benefits. Flaxseeds are a nutritional powerhouse: Filled with vitamins A and E, as well as fatty acids, they can work wonders for your skin whether you eat them or apply them to your face. So throw these powerful seeds into a smoothie or this face mask.

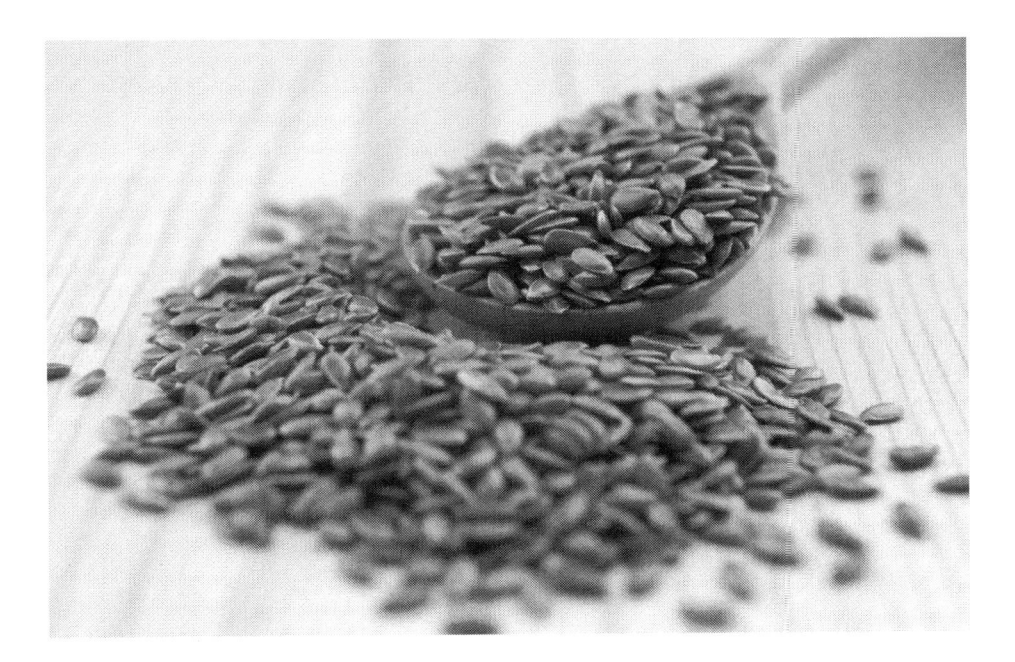

Ingredients
1 teaspoon flaxseed meal
3 teaspoons almond milk

Preparation
1. Soak the flaxseed meal in the almond milk until it reaches a gooey consistency, about 15 minutes.
2. Use immediately.

Storage
1. This recipe only makes enough for 1–2 uses, because soaked flaxseeds may not hold up well over time.

Directions for Use
1. Apply to dry skin.
2. Let set for 10 minutes or until the mask has dried.
3. Rinse off in circular motions.
4. This mask should leave your face feeling moisturized, but feel free to follow with an all-natural toner and moisturizer. You can also carry on with your normal skincare routine if you'd like.

Matcha Mask

Matcha green tea is packed with antioxidants that reduce inflammation and the signs of aging. Whether you drink it or apply it directly to your face, matcha just might be your anti-aging secret weapon.

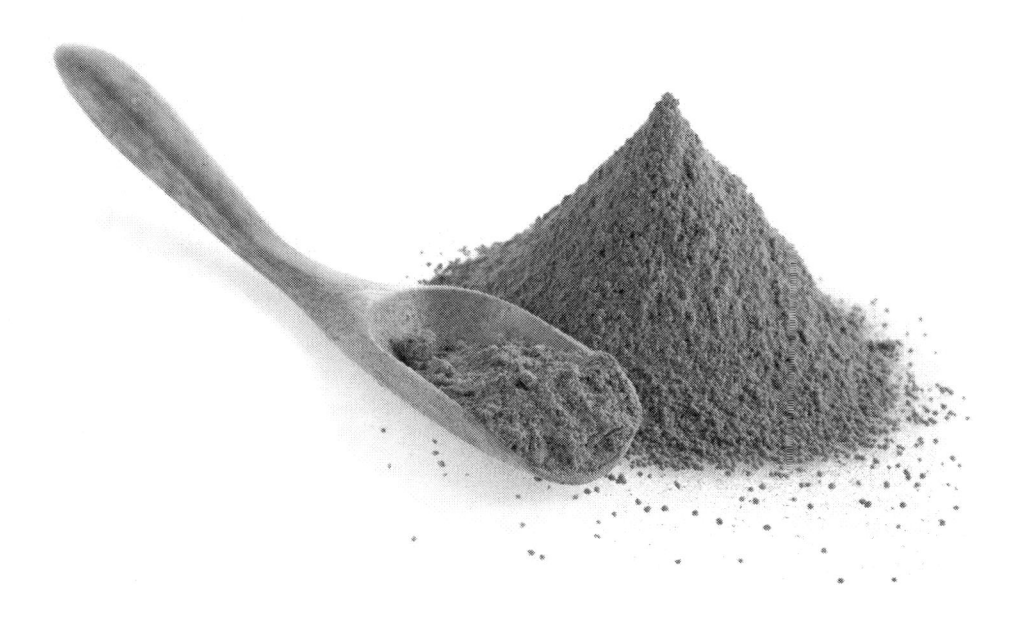

Ingredients
2 tablespoons matcha powder
1½ tablespoons aloe vera gel

Preparation
1. Mix ingredients together and scoop into an airtight container.

Storage
1. Store in an airtight container in the refrigerator for up to one month.

Directions for Use
1. Apply to dry skin.
2. Let set for 10 minutes or until the mask has dried.
3. Rinse off in circular motions.
4. This mask should leave your face feeling moisturized, but feel free to follow with an all-natural toner and moisturizer. You can also carry on with your normal skincare routine if you'd like.

Spirulina Mask

Spirulina and activated charcoal both have intense detoxifying properties, while spirulina is packed with antioxidants. That makes this mask an unbeatable combination.

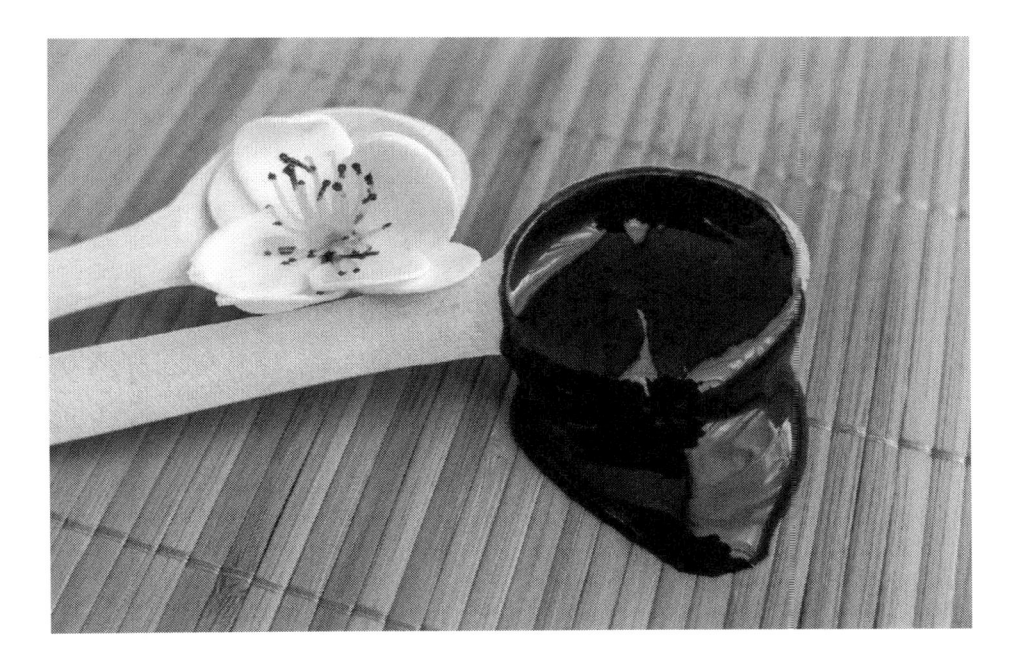

Ingredients
½ teaspoon spirulina powder
½ teaspoon activated charcoal
3 drops lavender essential oil
ACV (as needed)

Preparation
1. Combine all ingredients, adding apple cider vinegar as needed until you have a smooth paste.
2. Use immediately.

Storage
1. This recipe only makes enough for one use, because activated charcoal will dry out in the refrigerator.

Directions for Use
1. Apply to dry skin.
2. Let set for 10 minutes or until the mask has dried.
3. Rinse off in circular motions.
4. This mask should leave your face feeling cleansed, but feel free to follow with an all-natural toner and moisturizer. You can also carry on with your normal skincare routine if you'd like.

Chocolate Mask

Raw cocoa powder and pomegranates are both incredibly high in antioxidants, so this mask is a good choice for aging skin.

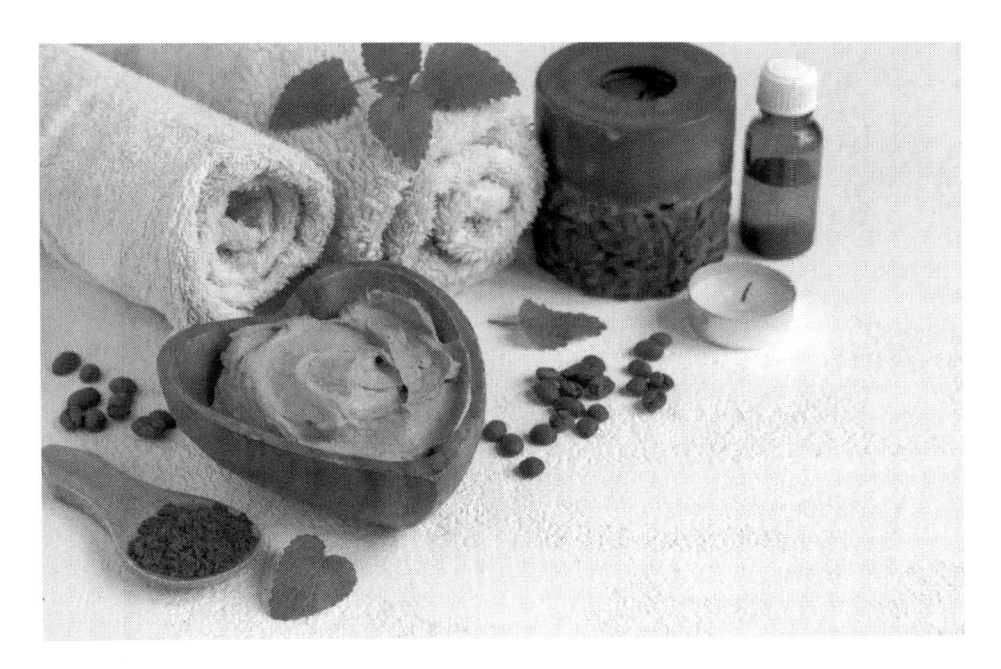

Ingredients
1 tablespoon raw cacao powder
3 drops pomegranate seed essential oil
Almond milk (as needed)

Preparation
1. Combine all ingredients, adding almond milk as needed until a paste forms.
2. Scoop into an airtight container.

Storage
1. Store in an airtight container in the refrigerator for no longer than one week.

Directions for Use
1. Apply to dry skin.
2. Let set for 10 minutes or until the mask has dried.
3. Rinse off in circular motions.
4. Feel free to follow with an all-natural toner and moisturizer. You can also carry on with your normal skincare routine if you'd like.

Avocado Mask

The naturally occurring oils in avocado make this mask super-moisturizing and nourishing, while aloe vera gel heals. This mask is perfect for chronically dry skin. Take that, winter dryness!

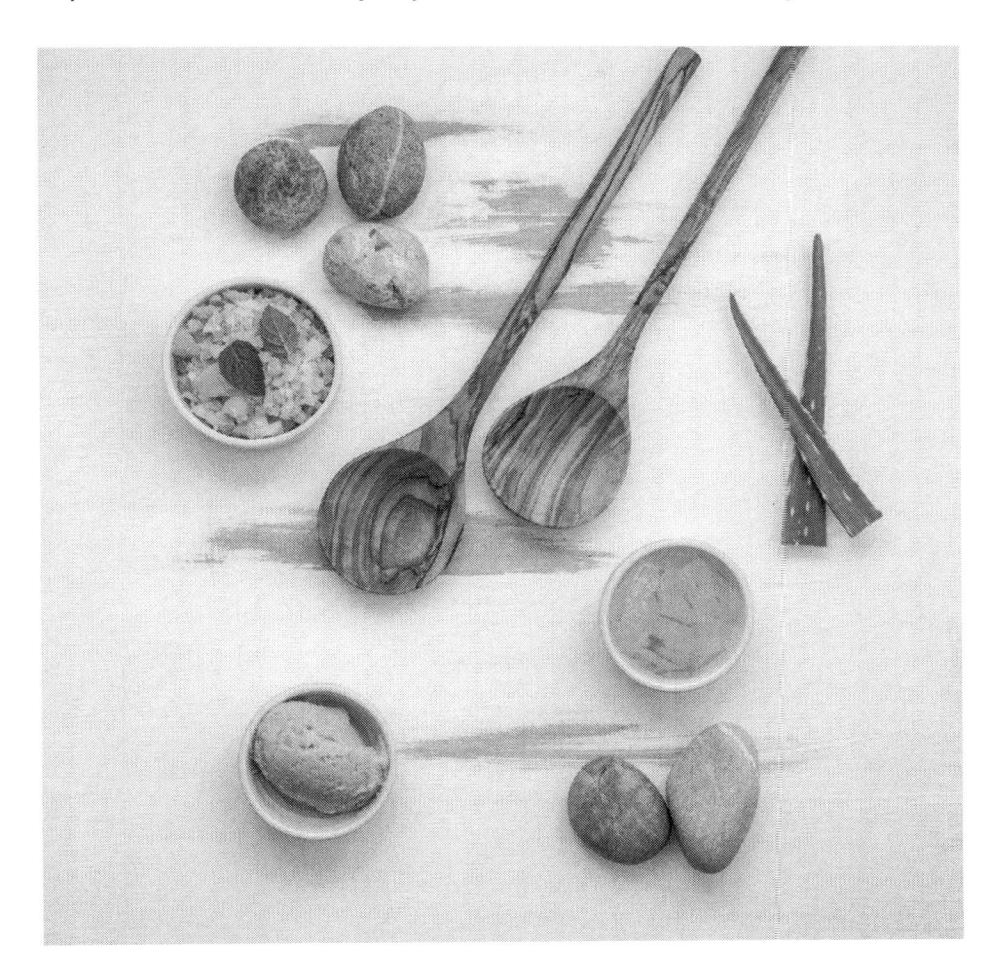

Ingredients
¼ avocado, mashed
1 teaspoon lemon juice, fresh
½ teaspoon spirulina
½ teaspoon aloe vera gel

Preparation
1. Mix all ingredients together.
2. Use immediately.

Storage
1. You may have noticed that avocado does not stand the test of time even if refrigerated, so use this mask immediately. If you have any leftovers, share with a friend or use on your body.

Directions for Use
1. Apply to dry skin.
2. Let set for 10–15 minutes.
3. Rinse off in circular motions.
4. This mask should leave your face feeling moisturized, but feel free to follow with an all-natural toner and moisturizer. You can also carry on with your normal skincare routine if you'd like.

Extras

Lavender Makeup Remover

This makeup remover is so simple, effective, and moisturizing, plus it has soothing essential oils that can help you sleep, making it a perfect addition to your nightly routine. Sleep well!

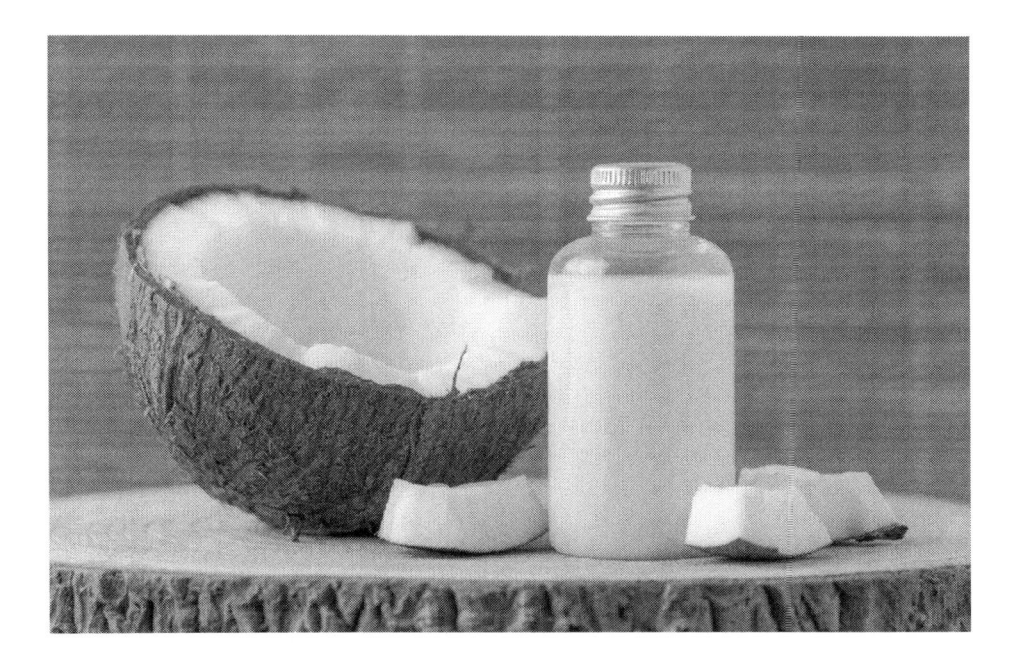

Ingredients
½ cup coconut oil
5 drops lavender essential oil
2 drops Roman chamomile essential oil

Preparation
1. Mix ingredients together and scoop into an airtight container.

Storage
1. Store in an airtight container.
2. Since coconut oil will sometimes harden if it is cold out, it's best to store this in a jar with a wide lid so you can scoop into it if necessary.

Directions for Use
1. Rub onto face with a cotton pad as needed until all makeup is removed. Follow with your normal skincare routine.

Coconut Oil Sunscreen

The key to flawless skin as you age? Sun protection! This sunscreen has no harmful ingredients, but all of the protection you need.

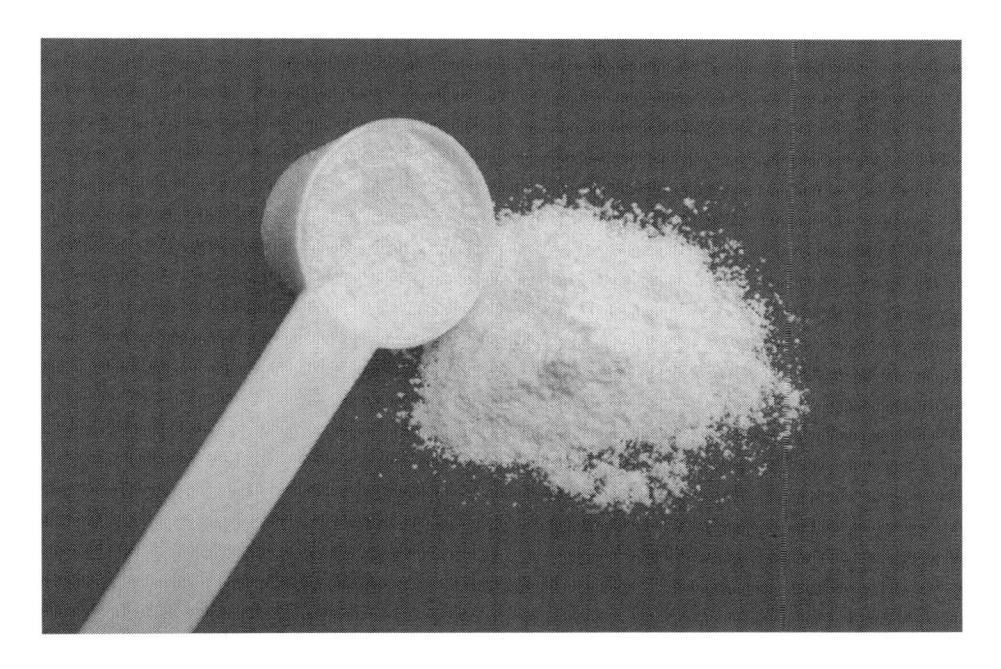

Ingredients
1 cup coconut oil
4 tablespoons zinc oxide powder
10 drops carrot seed oil

Preparation
1. Mix ingredients together and scoop into an airtight container.

Storage
1. Store in an airtight container.
2. Since coconut oil will sometimes harden if it is cold outside, it is best to store this in a jar with a wide lid so you can scoop into it if necessary.

Directions for Use
1. Apply to your face and entire body 30 minutes before sun exposure. Rub in well.
2. Reapply every 1–2 hours.

Cucumber Face Mist

Cucumber water is soothing for the skin and helps reduce under-eye puffiness. Add in the moisturizing benefits of coconut water, and this face mist is the perfect way to perk up your skin.

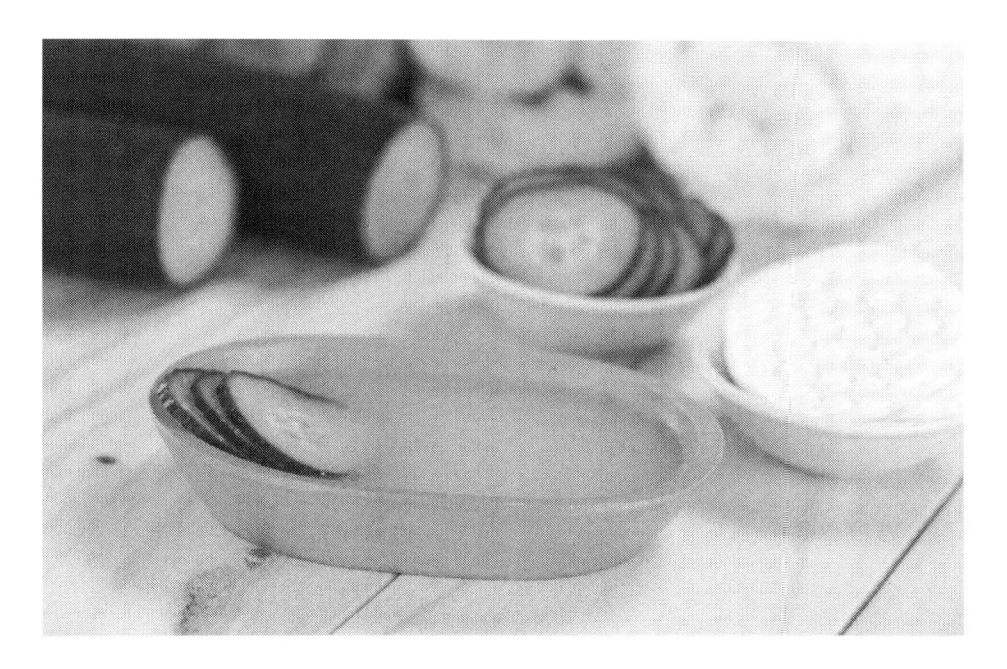

Ingredients
1 cup water
1 small cucumber, cleaned and diced
¼ cup coconut water

Preparation
1. Add the water and diced cucumber to a pan. Simmer for 5 minutes.
2. Strain out the cucumber pieces and add the water to a spray bottle with coconut water.

Storage
1. Store in the refrigerator no longer than you would normally store diced cucumbers, no longer than three days.
Haven't used it all after three days? Go ahead and drink it!

Directions for Use
1. Spray on clean skin when feeling tired or dehydrated.

Anti-Aging Frankincense Night Oil

Frankincense is one of the most powerful essential oils you can have in your routine. Together with argan oil, it smells amazing and makes a killer anti-aging oil.

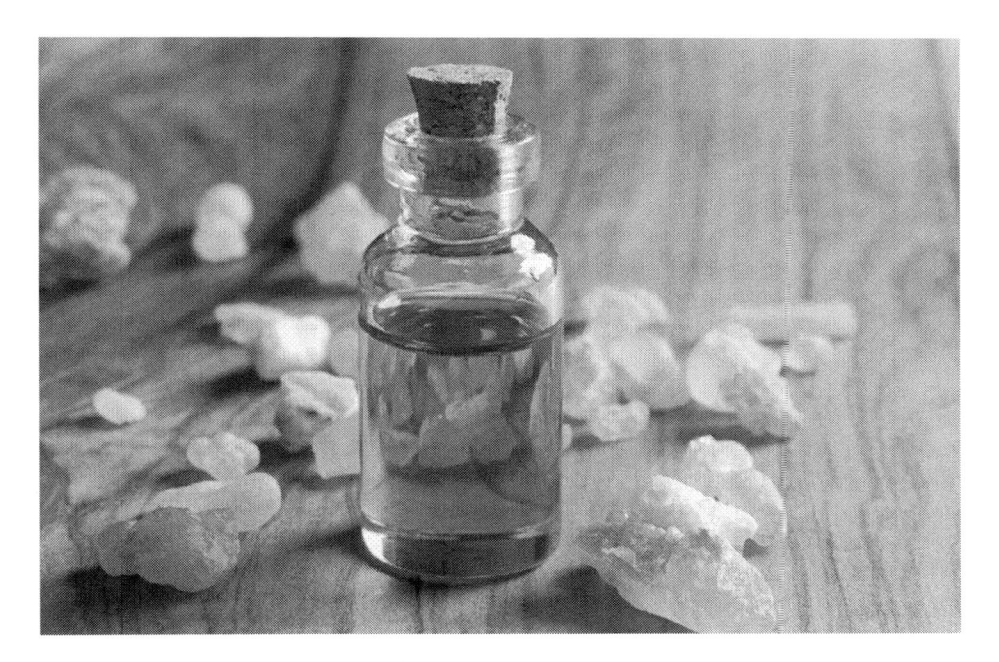

Ingredients
2 tablespoons argan oil
4 drops frankincense essential oil
2 drops bergamot essential oil
1 drop sandalwood essential oil

Preparation
1. Mix ingredients together and pour into an airtight container.

Storage
1. Store in an airtight container.

Directions for Use
1. Add a few drops to your moisturizer, or rub a few drops into skin at the end of your skincare routine.

Vanilla Lip Scrub

This lip scrub will keep chapped lips moist and smooth in the winter. Plus, it tastes and smells delicious!

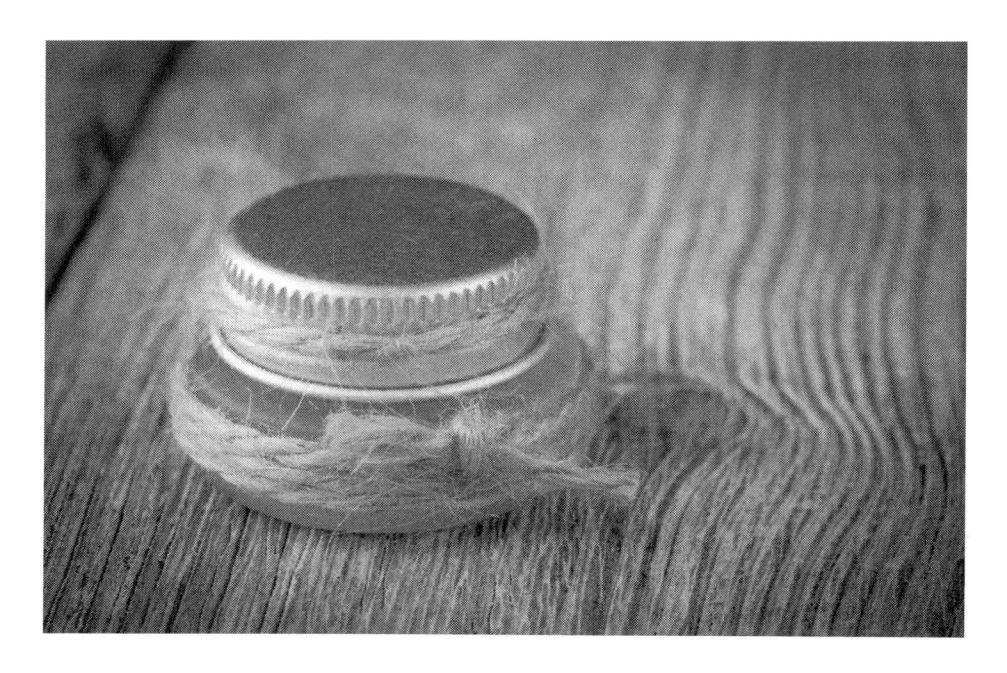

Ingredients
1 tablespoon coffee grounds, fresh
½ tablespoon jojoba oil
1 teaspoon shea butter
¼ teaspoon Vanilla Absolute

Preparation
1. Mix ingredients together and scoop into an airtight container.

Storage
1. Store in an airtight container for up to 2 weeks. No need to refrigerate.

Directions for Use
1. Rub into dry lips until satisfied.
2. Rinse off and follow with an all-natural lip balm or lip oil.

Argan Aftershave Balm

Men and women both suffer from irritated skin and red bumps after shaving. Not with this balm! The frankincense creates a sensual, gender-neutral fragrance anyone can enjoy.

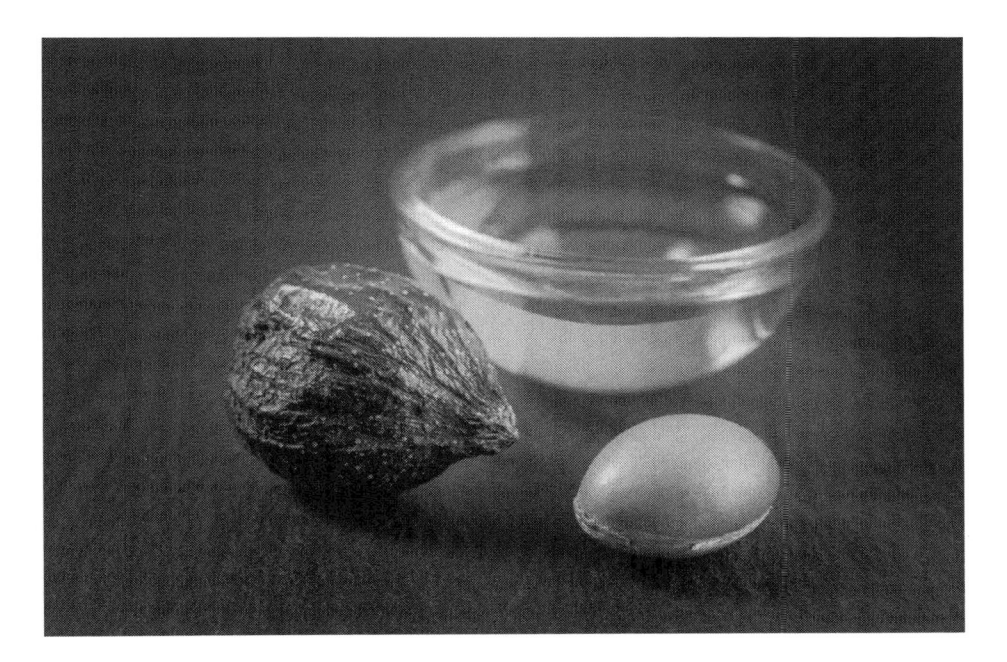

Ingredients
3 tablespoons shea butter
2 tablespoons argan oil
1 tablespoon aloe vera gel
5 drops frankincense essential oil
2 drops Roman chamomile essential oil

Preparation
1. Melt the shea butter and allow to cool slightly.
2. Mix in argan oil and aloe vera gel.
3. Once it has cooled completely, stir in the essential oils.
4. Scoop into an airtight container.

Storage
1. Store in an airtight container in the refrigerator for up to a month.
2. Leave out for 1–2 hours before use to let the shea butter soften.

Directions for Use
1. Apply a small amount to skin after shaving. No need to rinse off.

Super-Soothing Aftershave

This aftershave will prevent red bumps while providing essential oils that are soothing to the skin and mind. Storing in the refrigerator makes this aftershave even more soothing, plus the fragrance is gender neutral. Win-win-win.

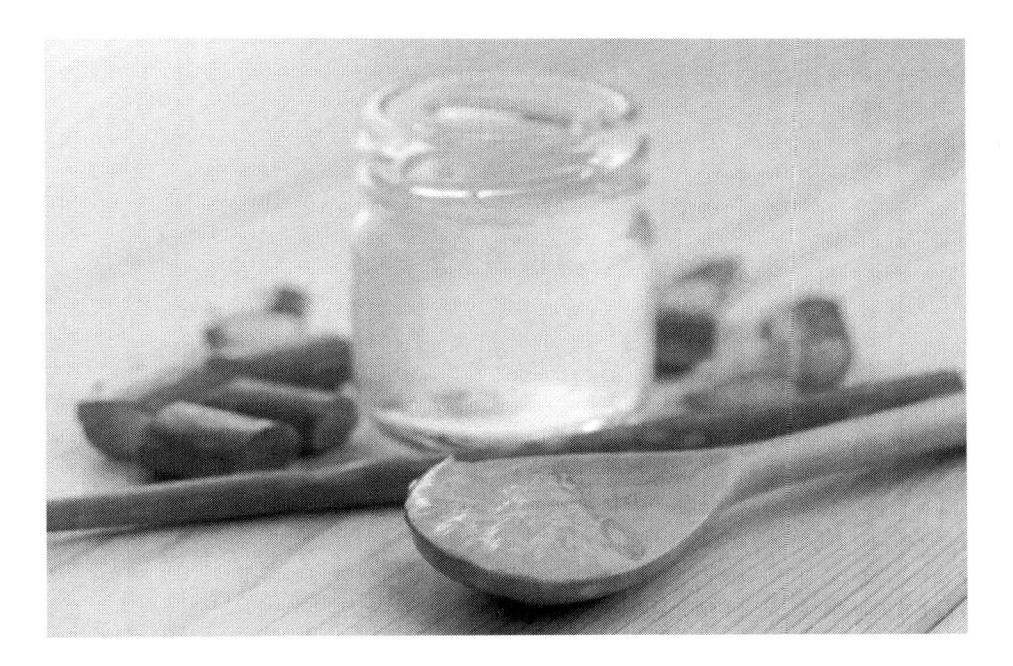

Ingredients
½ cup witch hazel
½ cup aloe vera juice
10 drops sandalwood essential oil
5 drops lavender essential oil
2 drops vetiver essential oil
1 drop clary sage essential oil

Preparation
1. Mix all ingredients together and pour into an airtight container.

Storage

1. Store in an airtight container in the refrigerator for up to a month. A spray bottle is a good option.

Directions for Use

1. Apply a small amount to skin after shaving. No need to rinse off.
2. The witch hazel may sting slightly if you have cut yourself. This is normal and not a cause for concern, but do not knowingly apply this product to open wounds.

Spot Treater

Evening primrose oil is said to balance hormonal acne, while manuka oil will dry out and heal blemishes. Aloe vera gel likewise delivers the healing damaged skin needs.

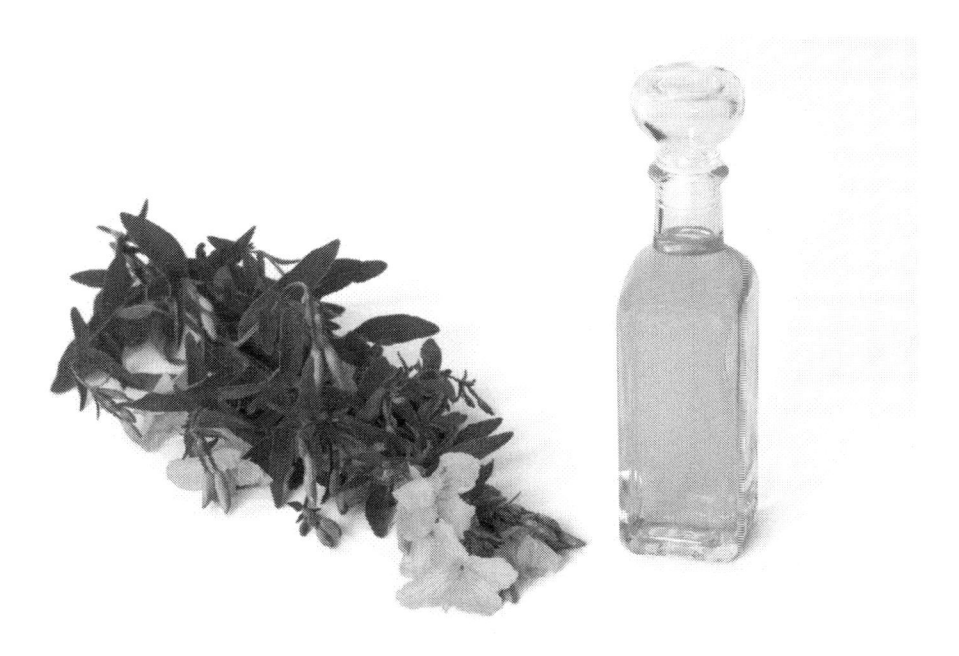

Ingredients
1 tablespoon evening primrose oil
1 tablespoon aloe vera gel
10 drops manuka oil

Preparation
1. Mix ingredients together and pour into an airtight container.

Storage
1. Store in an airtight container in the refrigerator for up to one month.

Directions for Use
1. Apply directly to pimples after you have finished your daily skincare routine. Perfect to use before bed.

Further Reading

Country wisdom & know-how: everything you need to know to live off the land. New York: Black Dog & Leventhal Publishers, 2004.

Donnelly, Chris. "DIY organics, medicinal herbs, organic beauty recipes, homemade face cream, and DIY all-natural." January 01, 1970. Accessed July 21, 2017. http://homemadeorganics.blogspot.com/.

Gray, Nicole. "DIY Organic Make-Up Recipes." Small Footprint Family. July 05, 2017. Accessed July 21, 2017. https://www.smallfootprintfamily.com/diy-organic-makeup-recipes.

Keville, Kathi. *Aroma therapy*. Lincolnwood, IL: Publications International, 1999.

Mama, Katie – Wellness. "How to Make Natural Makeup at Home." Wellness Mama. June 2, 2017. Accessed July 21, 2017. https://wellnessmama.com/4948/natural-makeup-recipes/.

"Natural Skin Care Archives." Coconuts & Kettlebells. Accessed July 21, 2017. http://coconutsandkettlebells.com/category/skin-care/.

Sruthika and Gnanika. "Health & Beauty." DIY Natural Home Remedies. Accessed July 22, 2017. http://diyremedies.org/.

Worwood, Valerie Ann. *The complete book of essential oils and aromatherapy*. San Rafael, CA: New World Library, 1991.

Also by Josephine Simon

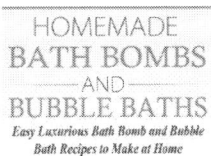

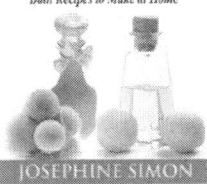

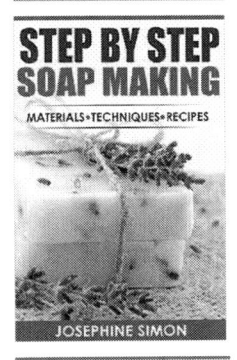

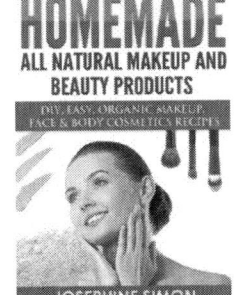

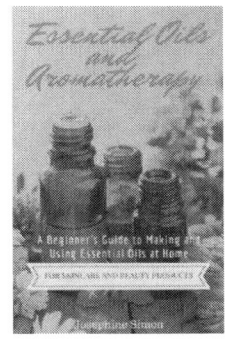

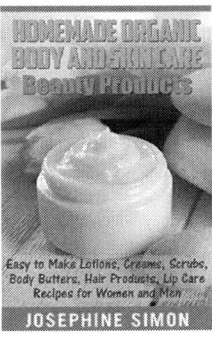

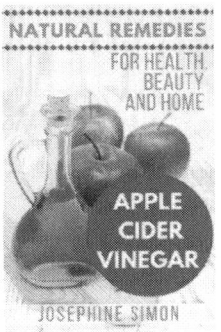

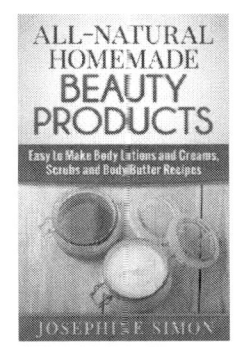

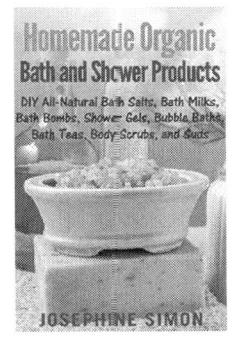

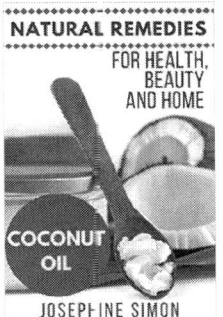

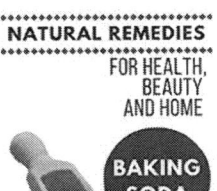

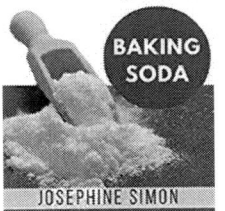

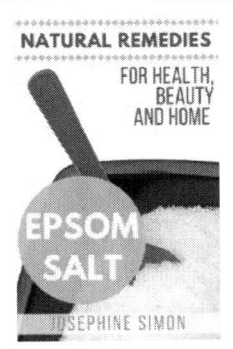

Printed by Amazon Italia Logistica S.r.l.
Torrazza Piemonte (TO), Italy